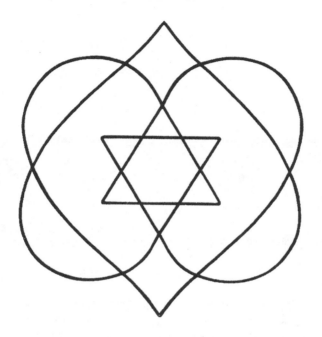

RIGHT USE OF WILL

Healing and Evolving
the Emotional Body

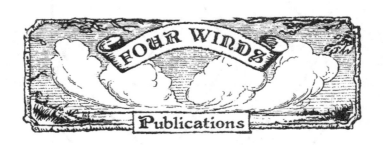

Copyright © 1984, 1986, 2010, Ceanne DeRohan
All rights reserved, including the right to reproduce this
book or any portions thereof in any form whatsoever without
written consent by the copyright holder.
For information address:
Four Winds Publications
1000 Cordova Pl. #112
Santa Fe, New Mexico, 87505
USA

These books are printed with soybean inks on recycled paper
and are not coated with plastic.

RIGHT USE OF WILL

Healing and Evolving
the Emotional Body

Received by Ceanne DeRohan

FOUR WINDS PUBLICATIONS

Dedicated to
the Earth

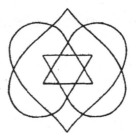

TABLE OF CONTENTS

INTRODUCTION

If this book is for you, you will know it from these first few pages. This book may stir emotional response. Please realize that this book is meant to trigger you and is not meant to be just a mental exercise. If you feel emotions being stirred, please do your best to allow these emotions direct expression as any sounds they want to make. Please do not act in response to what is being triggered; just be present with your emotions.

The unconditional love of the Spirit for everything that exists has been understood on Earth for quite some time. This, in fact, has been called Divine Love. Now there is need for another understanding on Earth – that of Divine Will.

Most people on Earth have made a separation between their Spirit and their Will. They have believed their own Will was not acceptable and that to love in the way that God loves, they must eliminate their own feelings and opinions and do what they have imagined to be the Will of God. An understanding is needed here: The Will of God is not in opposition to the Will of the individual.

Because of the separation that has been made in the consciousness of so many, the Will has been excluded for a long time from participating in the evolvement of the Spirit. A definite lag, or gap, exists on Earth between the level of evolvement of the Individual Spirit, often referred to as the Soul, and the evolvement of the Individual Will. It is now time for each Spirit to recognize, accept and evolve this other part of the self. Each Spirit is a part of God's Spirit, and each Will is a part of God's Will.

Each person must take responsibility for his or her complete being and not for only a part of it. The Will expresses Itself as feelings, emotions, receptivity, intuition and desire. Each Spirit must fully accept Its own Will and help It evolve in a loving way that is not punitive, judgmental or condescending. When the Individual Will feels that It truly has the loving acceptance of the

Spirit, It will be able to come into alignment with the Spirit and with the Divine Will.

God has given each individual a part of His Divine Consciousness with which to have awareness and a part of His Divine Will to feel what this awareness is experiencing. Everyone now wishing to remain on Earth must accept the whole being and discontinue denial of the part of the self that feels what the Spirit is experiencing.

Instead of denying your own Will in favor of someone else, or in favor of what you have believed to be the Divine Will, it is necessary, now, to realize that denial of the Individual Will has been a misunderstanding that has resulted in a split in the consciousness of individuals on Earth. The Individual Will is not meant to be separate from the Divine Will any more than the Individual Spirit is meant to be separate from the Divine Consciousness. It is important to realize this thoroughly and profoundly.

I received these words directly from God. In the beginning, I could not, like so many others on Earth, believe it was actually possible to hear directly from God. I knew, though, that many psychics have been accustomed to hearing from spirit guides. I found this to be very interesting, and I began to listen and learn from guides who had identified themselves to me as The Ancient Ones. As this went on, I was encouraged to try to hear directly from God. When I first heard Him, I was overcome with feelings of His exquisite love. I had been living without conscious awareness of this connection for so long that I hadn't realized how much I had been missing God and how much I was missing a strong feeling of His presence on Earth.

God wants it to be known that He is open and willing to communicate directly with all Spirits on Earth who can open to receive Him. When you are truly open and receptive to His Loving Light, you can begin to experience a direct communication. As you become more attuned, anything you need to know is then available because of the connection we all have with God.

God has given me the information in this book, and although He refers to Himself as God in these first paragraphs, now that this has been stated, He is going to refer to Himself as My Light or My Loving Light, and occasionally as I, in the rest of the text.

The Will has long been misunderstood because the Spirit was seen to be the essence of the Body, but the understanding is this:

Spirit inspires, Will responds and together They experience in the Body. Body is the manifestation of both Spirit and Will. In order for unconditional love to manifest in the Body, Spirit and Will must balance in the Heart. To find this balance, you will need to open the consciousness of your Spirit and the receptivity of your Will to receive My Loving Light.

My Light is polarized in order to experience. This polarization has been misunderstood as splits in which the Will was seen as disconnected from, and not a useful part of Spirit and has even been judged to be in opposition to the Spirit. However, the Spirit and the Will are the expanding polarities of Oneness. Polarities need to be recognized as evolving expansions of a connected whole.

Creation exists because it has both the Spiritual Essence that powers it and the Magnetic Energy that can open space to receive it. The same is true within each individual. The Spirit and the Will are not meant to be separate from one another in any individual any more than My Spirit is meant to be separate from My Will. In each person, the Spirit and the Will are meant to be unconditionally connected to each other. Each Individual Spirit is meant to be connected to My Spirit and each Will connected to My Will, and, so, all is One.

The understanding needed next is: When anything is denied and not accepted by the individual to whom it belongs, that denied part of the individual has been placed outside of his or her love. In placing something outside of love, you have been feeding another reality that has troubled Earth for a long time. Because of its negative polarity, most people have equated the Will with evil and with darkness. Everything negative has been assumed to be the cause of the trouble on Earth. You need to realize that this is not true.

Darkness and negativity need to be understood and accepted as the part of Creation that can make a place for My Light by opening the space to receive it. Until It opens space to attract and receive Light, the Will appears to be darkness. When the Will is not allowed to express, It cannot vibrate. It is the Will's vibration that opens space.

Now many people have thought they were evolving into unconditional love on Earth, but they have forgotten that they must accept all of themselves first. There is no way around it. If you do not totally accept yourself first, you cannot totally open to anyone or anything else. Many have thought that by allowing their Will to express only positive feelings, they would attract only Loving Light, but what they have attracted is the conditional love that results from denial.

Because the Will has been so misunderstood, the need to allow the Will to evolve is great right now on Earth. To evolve It, you must first accept It. You cannot beat It into the appropriate shape. It must be accepted as It is now in order to evolve. Denial of unlovingness will not clear It. You cannot just mentally insist that you are all loving. You must really be there. All levels of your being must really be there. Where your Will has not been allowed to open and receive Loving Light, you have denial. Your denials are yours to heal. In healing your Will, you must allow It to tell you how upset It has become. In hearing from your Will unconditionally, you have taken the step of accepting It, wherever It is.

Denial does not allow Loving Light in. Controlling and imposing limits and conditions on your Will means you do not have unconditional acceptance for It. Where you do not have acceptance for It, you are not loving It. Where you are not loving It, you are denying It. When you deny parts of yourself, you are not accepting all of yourself, and, so, you do not have all of yourself present with you. If you do not have all of yourself present with you in loving acceptance, you are not loving yourself unconditionally. You cannot love anyone or anything else unconditionally if you do not have all of yourself with which to love them. You must accept all of yourself unconditionally by bringing all parts of yourself within loving acceptance and allowing them to evolve.

When a person is denying parts of the self, that person will be denying others, too. No one who wants to continue on the path of self-denial or of denying others, (a path of imbalance, in other words), will be able to remain on Earth. It is not a loving, nourishing, life-giving policy to be living in a state of imbalance, but in saying this, a threat is not intended. Major spiritual misunderstandings have been in place from the very beginning and have beleaguered Earth from the beginning. This information is meant to help you understand how to release yourself from the path of strife, struggle and suffering that denial has brought to Earth.

Earth has been imbalanced to the point of feeling her life is threatened, and is not going to tolerate any more imbalance. The Earth, herself, is going to clear out of herself, and off of herself, everything that has not been loving toward her. As she is doing this, all those who want to remain on Earth must also clear out of themselves everything that has not been loving.

The understandings you need now are about how to help and allow your own Will to evolve. In short, allow your Will to express everything you feel, and do not stop until you are really finished. The problem with the free expression of the Will on Earth right now is that it has been denied for so long that its attempts to express itself have looked out of balance, and they often have been. For this reason, let your Will release in a private place, as the Will naturally would with sounds, especially at first. The emotional release My Light is talking about is direct emotional expression as sounds, so, be careful not to hurt yourself or anyone else, and do not go forward and act out on a wave of emotions.

In reading this book and trying out these understandings, it is important not to impose this on others who do not want it, for just as it is not spiritual balance to deny yourself in favor of others, it is also not spiritual balance to deny others in favor of yourself. It is also not necessary to believe that you must have teachers or intermediaries to help you find the healing you need. While others can have help to offer, you are the one who knows, and can know, yourself best. Take responsibility for yourself and what you need to do to heal your imbalances. While emotional release has been a long-neglected part of this healing process, understanding must also enter in where denial was, acceptance must take the place of non-acceptance and openness must come where you were closed. Your Will has a progression that can help you if you can allow it to unfold. You can also ask My Loving Light to help you.

Denial does not allow the release back out of what has been taken in. When you take in and do not release back out, your receptive centers get filled up and can no longer receive clearly, and sooner or later, not at all. Blocking the free expression of the Will has not been allowing the release back out of what the Will has taken in. This makes it very difficult to exercise discernment and is one of the main reasons that most people on Earth do not, at present, have direct experience of My Presence.

Much of what has shut down evolution of consciousness on Earth is fear, held in common by many, that free expression will result in harm to others, societal chaos or both. This fear is accompanied by another fear that so many who have claimed Divine Authority have done harmful things, and many who have claimed to hear Divine Impulses have done the bidding of voices that have told them to do harmful things. You can be sure that these claims of Divine Guidance are not My Loving Light if they have influenced people to do harmful things.

One of the empowering factors in these understandings is that you can release yourself intentionally by allowing free expression. This, then, eliminates the need for any harmful situation to come to you from outer reality. This is an understanding that is very necessary now on Earth. People have thought that karma brings a balance of payments, but karma is not that simplistic. Karma is meant to bring you into balance, this is true, but not by bringing one experience as payment for another in the past. Karma brings balance by attracting the experiences you need in order to learn what you do not yet know.

Without Will, the Spirit has no selection process. Your Will is your individual magnetic energy field and draws the experiences you are going to have. If you hold something in your Will that is denied and disconnected from your conscious awareness by not being accepted and allowed free movement or free expression, you will then draw a reflection of this to yourself. Unpleasantness is not sent by My Loving Light as punishment for misdeeds. Unpleasantness is only drawn in response to what has been denied or judged against. The denial is what gives the experience its unpleasant qualities.

The energy locked up in denial does not want to be held outside of the nourishment of Loving Light. In coming to you, drawn by the denial, unpleasant experiences have not come to punish. They have come to draw your attention to the denials. They are drawn to you in an attempt to release the energy that is being held there, outside of your loving acceptance. By allowing yourself to be easily triggered into releasing your held denials, the intensity of these reflections can lessen until you no longer need to draw to yourself any unpleasantness. Try it before you judge it.

Some of you can help each other by doing group release work if you have an agreement with one another about what is happening there. By allowing yourselves to express your boundaries and draw definite guidelines according to what you feel is necessary, you may be able to helpfully re-enact traumatic experiences in order to trigger yourself to release them. Because many people have received harm at the hands of others and have not yet released or expressed the pain of this, some may want, or need, the help of being triggered by others acting as though they are going to do harm. If you try this approach, only do what is needed to trigger the emotional release that will relieve the person; do not cause additional pain.

I also want to say that you can still take the path of letting experience come to you from without and balance yourself in that way. If you want to, in fact, you can even call for the karmic experiences necessary so that you can be triggered to release your own denial. Pleasant experiences will still happen, My Light is just addressing unpleasant ones right now. As you lessen and eliminate denial, you can create even more pleasant experiences and better ones. By shifting the power from a state of externalized disconnection to internalized conscious acceptance, you can always know what is going to happen. You might not have complete detail because you might have the kind of Will that likes surprises, but you will know it will be pleasant. This can give great peace to everyone.

My Light has been compelled to impart Right Use of Will to Earth at this time because the situation there has become very perilous. People on Earth, and even animals, because of being confined and controlled, have not been expressing freely enough to adequately vibrate their space and hold it open for themselves. My created beings on Earth have been experiencing their reality as seeming to close in on them, and their power as seeming to be insufficient to meet the situation facing Earth now. Please realize it does not have to be this way; the lost light of misunderstandings and denial of the Will have made it this way. If you want to be able to live on Earth, you must now start reversing the situation within yourself. It is not going to be easy at first, but it will become easier the longer you work on it.

My guidance is to preserve the balance points that provide the most freedom for everyone without eclipsing anyone, and are necessary to maintain Spirits and the Creation in which they live. Earlier, it was apparent to Me that many Spirits could not accept My Guidance because they did not have enough experience to understand why these balance points were so important. I have seen that the Spirits on Earth now have had enough experience to be able to accept, understand and respect these balance points, and so, I want to make it clear that I am decisive on several points where I was open to allowing Spirits to transgress earlier. These decisions are decrees.

All Spirits wishing to remain on Earth must recognize Me and come to Me for Loving Light. No Spirit can continue to deny Me and take My Light underhandedly from others.

Now, in physical Body, the reality of this is one thing and one thing only. No one can survive anymore in My Creation unless they acknowledge Me and accept My Loving Light openly in some form. I am flexible here. I have many ways to come to a Spirit. I can adjust Myself infinitely, but I will no longer tolerate complete denial of Me any place in My Creation. This means that no Spirits can survive what is happening now, any place in My Creation, unless they open to directly receive My Loving Light. You must not think you are not involved if you accept Me as God and worship Me. You must find your denials, bring them within your love and find them acceptable to Me.

I am not being unloving or unmerciful here. If I am unlimited, and I am, I can no longer tolerate Spirits who want to limit Me to the extent of being in My Creation and refusing to allow Me to be there with them. I have said this to give you the opportunity to reverse your own denials. If you feel a need to critique this message or attack Me for what is not being said here, this is your pathway into the emotions you need to express in order to find out how you really feel about Me. I have many understandings to give on why I have made these decrees, but they are not appropriate to give right now. Trust that they will be given at the right time.

I have also made another decree. I have no further tolerance for any Spirits giving pain to others who have not overtly agreed to receive it. There has been such a thing as overriding of Free Will in the experience of My created Spirits. I have let this go on only long enough for the Spirits to see why the Will is so necessary. Now, I have discerned that there has been enough experience. There is no longer any power to override another's Will, period. Your own Will can only be overridden by your own denials. This has to be understood. Free Will between people means that you have the freedom to do whatever you want, but you are not to encroach on another or try to make anyone else function within your own limits. You only have the power to make them take it away from you or to take yourself away from them. There is no power anymore to stop anyone from experiencing themselves in the way they want to experience themselves. If you go against this, you are going against Me.

There is still some time on Earth for Spirits to show My Loving Light whether it is their intention to align with Me, or not. I have heard the cries of the Spirits who cannot handle anymore pain, control and unlovingness. I am offering the understandings needed for My Spirits to release themselves from the path of struggle, strife and suffering. Because there are still many who do not believe that this is My Loving Light talking here, they are going to have to learn from the experiences they create for themselves. I am going to put them in their right place. If you do not want to go with them, you need to find and recover your own lost Will and lost Light involvement in this.

In accepting these understandings, you only need to try them out, stop judging them and allow them to be in process. You will find that they work for you and everyone else who is ready to try them. Some on Earth have not yet had enough experience to try them, so I am reminding you again not to try to force these ideas on anyone. Just take them in if they are for you.

In studying this book, connect to the spirit of the message, and do not pass judgment on what has been left out. If there seems to be a gap that you cannot readily fill in with your logical, sequential thinking, you need to remain open, and trust that it will be given to you when you have the readiness to receive it. Many things that can be available to you through direct communication with My Loving Light have to be withheld from the public domain until the general population has more open acceptance. This is necessary also in order to protect and insure that those of you who choose to practice these teachings are not overloaded, since, at present, the mind is much more capable of quickly receiving these understandings than is the Will.

If you now temporarily stop the mental acquisition of this writing and give it time to sink into your feelings, you are going to have a response. If you do not have a response, then you have either lost your Will or you are not connecting to it. Some people have disconnected so much that they actually have to search out and find their missing Will. It is not impossible to do this. You can start by calling for it, if it's not present with you, and draw it back to you. Acceptance is the key once again. You must make a place for your Will.

If you are responding, let it happen and do not assume you have all the understandings needed. Allow your response and seek more understandings.

I now invite you to read, when you're ready, the rest of this book.

RIGHT USE OF WILL

The unconditional Love of the Spirit is understood by many people on Earth at present. There is another energy, though, that is also part of the Divine Creation, which has not yet been fully understood—the Divine Will.

The Will expresses as feelings. Spirit and Will are partners in the Body and must find their balance in the Heart. If there is any dis-ease or aging of the Body, Spirit and Will are at odds in some way. When there is balance in the Heart between the Spirit and the Will, Body manifests this internal balance as health, agelessness and vitality, and the physical level of existence is no longer experienced as cut-off from other levels of existence.

Everyone on Earth today has undermined the Will in some way. This undermining of the Will is equal to lost unconditional love, then, for anyone who is judging against parts of the self is not truly loving unconditionally.

The Will in many people is now seeking to find alignment. Many people on Earth can learn the balance of Spirit and Will in their Heart, and are, in fact, already moving in this direction. It could be easily judged then, that the teaching of *Right Use of Will* is not essential, and that this is just going to happen naturally. However, help with the understanding of this process is actually necessary, and some people want this help so that they can move faster. Others, who see little need to speed things up, can make the choice to find this alignment later. What may not seem necessary to you now, may become relevant at any moment.

This teaching is intended to be a guide for those who wish to speed up the process of finding the necessary balance between Spirit and Will in the Heart. The information given here may not all be new information to you, but it will outline the steps necessary to heal the disconnections and lack of self-acceptance so that balance with the Spirit can be willingly found. It can also enable you to see where you are on this path and can help you to go further.

CLEARING ILLNESS AND HABITS

To begin with, illness can be cleared by learning to listen to and accept what Body is trying to say to you when you are ill. Understanding these messages, without subjugating your Body to pre-formed opinions, gives your Body a most needed feeling of acceptance in place of the feeling that it is you dominating and controlling your Body or that your Body is against you and that you must defeat or banish illness as though it is some kind of sabotage by your Body. Illness is not sabotage. It is the Body's statement that it is unable to continue holding blockages to My Loving Light and also maintain health.

Messages from your Body can take many forms. Your Body may want and need many different things. Attuning to and accepting these messages can help you to regain the balance that enables illness to disappear and health to prevail. This statement, however, does not mean that you need to heal everything without whatever help you feel you need, that you must go the entire way with the first illness that appears or blame yourself if this interaction with your Body is more than you feel able to master right away. Unconditional acceptance and love means accepting whatever state of imbalance you have with your Body and understanding it as the reflection you need in order to notice and heal your imbalances without judgment about how spiritually evolved you are or are not. Being conscientious and doing what you can each time will carry you toward balance.

A way to work with healing in this way, is to give the dis-ease your full attention by breathing into and bringing your consciousness into the distress rather than blocking it, ignoring it or masking it with medication. See if you can feel what is going on in this distress. Ask your Body what it needs to restore balance. You can encourage your Body to communicate by letting it know that you have acceptance for its pain. You can apologize to your Body for overriding and ignoring it. Becoming aware of beliefs you have been holding about your Body, and what it needs, and releasing them is another helpful part of any shifts you make in the way you have been treating your Body. When you receive information from your Body, do what is asked and see the results. If complete healing is not reached, you can repeat this process until healing is reached. This practice can evolve your ability to listen to your Body and to bring it the healing it needs.

When treatment seeks to cure by suppressing symptoms, balance is not truly restored. The practice of suppressing symptoms is not the way Body heals itself. The practice of ignoring how Body feels or taking drugs for pain can often obscure early symptoms so that the person is not aware of the problem until it is acute and advanced. These denials can allow the imbalances that produce dis-ease to go unnoticed until the symptoms have had to demand attention by becoming intense. Then, healing can take a tremendous amount of time, energy, concentration, dedication and also money. It is really much easier to pay attention to Body and deal with imbalances in the beginning stages, than to wait until your Body is seriously challenged. If balance can be restored while symptoms are still at subtle levels, dis-ease may not need to appear.

Modern science has been spending a lot of time and money searching for "the cure" for dis-eases, but has not usually identified the cause as internal, spiritual imbalance. Illness can provide opportunities for clearance of more than just physical symptoms. The need for this sort of clearance always gives warnings in some way. You can help yourself by paying attention to how you feel about having to interrupt what you have been doing in order to respond to warning signals. Most people, though, have had a habit of ignoring such warnings, and also of suppressing symptoms, until the Body is holding so much that symptoms are only the tip of the iceberg of undermined Will.

Lack of loving acceptance for parts of the self originates every imbalance that manifests in the Body. When these imbalances become more than the Body can handle, physical problems arise. This is when pathogens can multiply into illness. Denial creates energy blockages, and blockages create stagnation which can be hospitable to disease organisms. These blockages are places where My Loving Light is not very present or not present at all. Disease organisms have always been present as physical manifestations of denial. To find full healing, you need to find the cause, not only in your physical body, but also in your consciousness, or lack of it.

Symptoms can help you find their cause. If you want to receive and understand their messages in order to find full healing, symptoms should not be routinely relieved or suppressed. Treatments that only address symptoms do not bring a full healing; however, this does not mean that symptoms should never be treated. Treating symptoms while also seeking the cause is different from suppressing them so that you can ignore them and go on as you were before.

When imbalances manifest as physical problems, there are many feelings involved that need exploration. All of these feelings need unconditional acceptance; however, mentalizing feelings by only talking about them is not the way full healing is going to take place. The more you attune to and express from Will/Body in the ways They want and need to express, the more you will be able to clear before illness or unpleasant experiences manifest as an attempt to bring clearing.

Even though some dis-eases indicate drastic imbalance, the idea that certain diseases are fatal has been accepted by many only because the way of treating them has been to deny the message of the Body and treat Body like it is something to manipulate. Instead of seeking to restore the balance, this approach has attempted to suppress all symptoms. Then, Body is rendered incapable of healing. Body has its own free Will to decide if it can heal now or not. No person needs to die from illness if Body has another option that is real for it. If you are seriously trying to align, Body will not die unless it needs the option of rebirth for full healing.

Many people have felt guilty if they have begun to think that they have caused their own dis-ease. It is important to have self-acceptance for whatever form your lessons take and compassion for yourself for wherever you are on your path and for whatever you are able to evolve. Love and compassion coming in the place of old misunderstandings can bring healing. No matter how far you are able to progress toward full healing, continuing to seek the cause and working with your problems is a healing path.

When there is the balance needed for health, an individual's energy is freed to create something other than dis-ease. Health is an offering to Spirits who can understand the way to live in the physical plane on Earth. The other abilities of *Right Use of Will* are based on a foundation of good health, because a Body blocked by imbalance cannot express the capabilities inherent in balance. Health can be the permanent state of affairs when Spirit and Will balance unconditionally in the Heart. The practice of *Right Use of Will* may at first, however, bring forward illness because a suppressed Will is bound to have suppressed symptoms which Body has had to hold. If imbalance is not rectified, illness is "healed" only temporarily.

The fear with which society has surrounded illness and death is a conditioning in need of strong attention. So many people have come to feel that illness is inevitable and that all must die of something, that the energy field emanated by these deep-seated beliefs has actually been perpetuating itself through the acceptance of it as inevitable. Even though health is the way, it has not been the way for such a very long time on Earth that it has appeared as though no one any longer still believes that this really is the way.

More immediate than regaining health for some people, is the need to examine habits that are running the Body down. Another way to look at this is to make a choice between living as you are for a short time and living long if you are willing to grow and make the changes necessary for good health. Once again, this is a matter of personal choice.

Right Use of Will offers the opportunity of enjoying life to its fullest. This is what many people say they are doing when they indulge in habits. Habits appeal to memories of having felt good, but habits actually set the Body up for physical death. Habits are a problem because they override the sensitive response of Body to a particular situation, and instead, impose a ritualized behavior that a person has used in the past, whether the present calls for the same response or not. Response from habit precludes response that is attuned to the particular situation.

Habits are to the Body what judgments are to the awareness. Both have a rigidity. Habitual behavior is a judgment that what was called for once is also called for now, and, therefore, no growth or change has taken place. In the same way that judgments stop and control the evolution of the consciousness, habits stop and control the evolution of the Body. Just as all levels of the being are run down by rigidity that suppresses the vibration, Body is run down by the rigidity of habit patterns that lack sensitivity to its changing needs. The reasons for the habit need to be found and then accepted and understood, not condemned and disciplined away.

The Body and the Body's actions remain imbalanced unless the person is willing to respond to the true needs of the moment rather than taking a habit learned in the past and projecting it onto the present because it seems to apply. All habits need attention, for many, such as ways of breathing, making love, eating by the clock, reacting to situations without fully perceiving them first and also, habitual verbal responses can be easily overlooked.

Encouraging the self is more healing than forcing the self, holding the self back or suppressing the self. Dictatorship to end habits is another form of suppression. Habits can only really be released when the person is ready to see why the habit is there. All of the emotions and beliefs around the habit need to be accepted and allowed to express so that they can participate in the person's spectrum of awareness.

Body also needs to express its feelings about habits. If habits have been suppressing this communication, but intent is to end the habit of overriding parts of the self, letting habits lapse to find out what has been suppressed can be helpful. The feelings underneath habits are often feelings that are being denied by the person who is using habits in place of true response. Then, there is also present a habit of avoiding feelings. In this case, the person needs to look at the habit of avoiding feelings and decide if this is what he/she wants to continue doing or not. If all the feelings are allowed total acceptance and expression, they can begin to tell the person what is needed in place of the habit patterns.

All of the habits and appetites that people have thought they enjoyed have been judged against by various spiritual belief systems as harmful to spiritual development. Lists of things to avoid have included such things as alcohol, sugar, red meat or any animal products, drugs, caffeine, marijuana, tobacco, sexual enjoyment and extremes of any kind. An understanding needed here is that the problem has not been these things, themselves, so much as the habit patterns and extremes of imbalance that have been so often associated with them.

Substances have been thought to be causal, but it is consciousness that is causal and nothing else. For example, eating meat, and especially red meat, has long been thought to make people too dense to receive spiritual illumination and yet, it is not causal here. The desire and need to eat meat has accompanied the consciousness needing to eat it. As loss of vibratory rate increased on Earth, density of the physical plane increased. Nourishment must match the vibratory rate of the consciousness taking it in. In not understanding what was causal here, many judgments have been made, and many have tried to break out of habits, giving up meat for example, by using discipline and control. This method only causes the habit pattern to change its form.

Breaking out of habits may look like a stumbling block to many, but realizing the goal, and seeing habits for what they are, is going to allow the process through which they can drop away. The immediate goal is to free yourself emotionally, which will enable you to feel better, to be more free and to enjoy life more. Once you begin this path, you may find that the gratification of finding acceptance for parts of yourself that were formerly suppressed is gradually and steadily replacing your need for your habits.

Many people have thought that *Right Use of Will* is too difficult to do or means giving up habits in a spirit of sacrifice or self-denial, however, whatever you can do toward freeing your Will is not as difficult as living in a Body that has to hold the blockage, resistance, denial and rigidity of an imprisoned Will. This loss of vibration can produce intense symptoms in the Body which draws attention to these held places. Even though many have been intimidated by their symptoms and have felt they must take medicine to suppress them, this is also an opportunity to deeply connect to Body.

Feelings of being unable to receive Body's messages, or understand them adequately enough to balance the Body, are the result of a longstanding gap between Spirit, Will and Body. This gap will resolve with practice, and the feelings of fear will dissolve as success gives confidence to the process. If, at present, the fear is overpowering the ability to receive Body's messages and respond to them, reassurance can be sought from others. However, reassurance only helps if you also seek your own feelings here, rather than abdicate to another's reality.

Feelings of confidence and fear both need acceptance. They need to be allowed to bring understandings through the process they generate. Fear could be hidden in habitual dependency upon your helpers. The origin of the fear needs exploration and understanding. Do not judge in advance what the fear is. Feel the fear, and let it give you the understandings. Release of any block improves clarity. Clarity improves communication. When you really listen to yourself, you can heal yourself. Then you can seek help in the spirit of confidence, knowing you need and want the help you request, rather than being dependent and confused because you don't know yourself.

The undermining of free Will on Earth has been accompanied by another habit; the habit of looking outside the self for the answers. This habit has another aspect to it; that of denying your own Will in favor of someone else's idea of what is best for you. This imbalance has opened the way for rules and generalized procedure because no one really knows what each and every moment calls for in someone else.

This lack of attunement is a direct result of denying the Will its right place. Freeing of the Will to do what it is meant to do is going to return to each person the sensitive and appropriate attunement to the self and everything the self does. No amount of refining or improving standardized procedures, applied programs, rules, regulations or, for that matter, manners is ever going to come close to the individualized fine-tuning that free Will has to offer. Your Will is meant to guide you in this so that what is appropriate to any given situation is what you feel like doing and also do. When the Will has been suppressed, it cannot give clear guidance. It has become clouded by what it has had to hold. Habits are substitutions in the place of attunement and attempts to compensate for the loss of attunement.

Because of past denials, Will and Body may not, at first, trust the Spirit to be responsive and may not fully trust for quite some time. Since so many messages have been ignored in the past, some time and experience may be needed for Will and Body to believe that this pattern is really changing. If this is the case, it doesn't need to mean that you should give up. You can accept your feelings of wanting to give up and also continue on this path. Learning through experience gives the best understanding. At present, almost all individuals are holding conditions on this. Conditions limit growth in that they are judgments that can color perceptions of experience. Free Will allows the evolution that can learn from experience, while the rigidity of judgments and habits creates repetitive experiences. A person's experience is his/her own individually unique experience and may or may not be the same as anyone else's. Learning from your own experience allows each of you to evolve in your own way. Learning in this way doesn't preclude the acceptance of advice or the sharing of observations and insights, and it allows everyone to be free. Your Will needs to be allowed to recover and evolve with the rest of your being in order for you to experience and express the full gift of your spiritual presence on Earth.

The balance of Spirit and Will in the Heart can be attained and can produce the health in the Body that is the starting point for evolving in harmony with your outer reality. When there is balance, harmony and joy accompanying the way of evolving, physical existence can be as enjoyable as any other plane of existence and can evolve to include all possibilities. You are then able to do what you want to do when you want to be doing it and for no other reason than that it is what you truly feel like doing.

In the process of balancing, allow yourself to notice whatever attracts you. The Spirit can see all possibilities. The Will is meant to select what is right for the moment among the possibilities. The Will does this through its feelings. Unconditional acceptance of feelings, including receiving input from Body, then allows the maximum learning, evolvement and attunement. Everything that is experienced can be accepted as a part of the process you need in order to find this balance. As your Spirit and Will come into alignment, this increasing balance will allow you to see how predestination and free Will are not in conflict with one another because all people are destined to find the balance of free Will.

This is still a matter of personal choice, however. No one can make you free your Will, and yet, you cannot force your Will to be a prisoner indefinitely, either. If freeing your own Will feels like the path for you now, you are ready to do it. If you don't know, you can let free Will unfold. If you don't want to free your Will at this time, you can go on as you are and see how that really feels to you. Respect yourself here. There may be reasons that you are not ready. Respect for others is also necessary. Do not try to convince anyone else that they should take this path, have to take this path or do this now. The gift that free Will has to offer is for everyone, but at the time that feels right for each person.

LIMITS ON THE SELF

The next step in evolving your own spiritual presence is to accept all of the reality you were meant to have on Earth. In accepting this reality, unconditional acceptance of the feelings is necessary. Feelings are meant to balance the Spirit's overview with the Will's perception of what is pleasant and possible for any given moment. Finding this balance in the Heart creates a reality in which all needs can be met without overriding in any direction.

An attuned Will has the ability to take you anywhere you want to go and to feed you and keep you warm. Holding the condition, or judgment, that these things must be worked for is part of the reason the Will hasn't been able to provide these things in another way. Release of these limitations is an important part of being able to enjoy yourself in the physical plane without having to work at something you do not want to do. Remember also, that if the feeling in the Will is to rest for a while, this is alright, too.

Judgments against allowing yourself to do what you want to do need release, as these held beliefs participate in the creation of your own reality. The release of attitudes and opinions about what it takes to live on Earth can open the space for things to change for you. Old conditioning does not let you assess a situation for what it is. Old conditioning takes the role of keeping your responses the same. When you no longer want it, you can feel imprisoned by it and not know how to get out. Trying to escape by rearranging your thoughts is only partially successful. When you understand how to release old conditioning, present feelings can let you know if something is right for you or not.

Misunderstandings have placed a great burden of limiting beliefs upon the self. Longstanding conditioning layered onto these limitations has been diminishing human possibilities instead of expanding them. Many have continued to accept limitations on the self because these many layers of conditioning have convinced them of their reality, or of their necessity. Some have been seeing these limitations as if they are what defines them as a person. Many limitations have been disguised as truisms, such as "Jack of all trades, master of none," or even, "I am a mathematician," when this statement excludes other things, even subtly.

Limiting beliefs need to be lifted off of the self as you feel ready. Whether you presently have the words for them or not, these limitations take the form of judgments held against the self. Many of the judgments, or limitations, that you may not want to continue living within can be seen in your daily dialogue with yourself and others. What do you do, say and believe that has been keeping you in the prison of limitations on the self?

Expressing yourself freely is the way to call for the reality you want, and yet, desire has long been judged to be a sin. In fact, desire is magnetic energy of the Will. Magnetic energy attracts, so it is important that you give acceptance to your desire so that you can know what it is that you are attracting. Desire, including desiring something other than what has been happening to you, needs loving acceptance and understanding just like anything else that has been judged against and, thus, placed in a state of being denied.

Love can be present when you open the space for it, and love can manifest in many forms. Loving acceptance for everything is the Divine Plan for all, so there is no need to continue fearing that My Plan calls for anything else. Bondage to others, self-denial, sacrifice, strife, struggle, starvation and scarcity are not the way of Limitless Love. These are the manifestations of misunderstandings closing down the openings through which love can manifest until

10

love can even appear to be punishment. Other than the beliefs, limitations and judgments you have been holding against yourself, there is nothing to punish you.

Is it not logical, then, that Love will provide if it is allowed to, since this is Love's way? Feelings of being undeserving must be released also. Judging yourself to be more, or less, deserving than others is not being open to what is simply appropriate, which is what you are capable of receiving in any given moment. Feelings of superiority, or inferiority, are off balance. Unconditional love accepts all as perfect in the moment, and yet, love loves everything as it needs to be loved and as it can accept love, which also means that everything can also shift, change, grow and evolve.

The path of bringing the balance of Spirit and Will into your Heart will show you what is right for you, and you will be able to recognize the perfection of it as you move along. Finding your own right place is a reflection of finding your own inner balance. In other words, as you are finding your inner balance, your outer reality will match it. In freeing your own Will, you cannot help but have your outer reality respond. It will also reflect whatever you have not found in yourself that needs to be brought within your loving acceptance. The longer it takes; the more conditioning you have to work through.

Right Use of Will works if you know it is the path for you. The Will is more than ready to receive the Love and Light of the Spirit. It is the individual Spirits who must accept the question of free Will and decide if it is right time or not. The feeling that recovery and healing of the Will is too difficult is part of the illusion that has kept the physical plane of existence seemingly separate from the other planes of existence, or speeds of vibration. This belief has been involved in the immense loss of vibration in the Will, and goes along with the belief that gifts are the reward of much dedication and hard work. The release of these judgments is necessary. Many spiritual teachers have said this because they have believed in separations that are not real or because they are confused and have taken the path of struggle and punishment.

Attuning your Spirit and your Will can be accomplished if you have the intention to do it. Spiritual teaching should not be directing you to lift above and drop off the physical and emotional bodies in order to return to God, the Light, the Source or whatever it is being called, without Them. These are old misunderstandings that have placed many limitations on the self. The reality is that this approach will not work. What is yours is yours, and you cannot solve anything by dropping it off. The way is to evolve, and to evolve you must begin to accept all of yourself in whatever state it is in.

In the path of each person there is what is called "Original Cause." *Right Use of Will* is beginning with what you are able to accept at first, so that a foundation can be built for understanding how these spiritual misunderstandings originated. For now, all that can really be said is that it is not possible to return to essence by dropping off parts of the self. Undercurrent here, are judgments against Creation.

Manifested Creation is not to be denied or gotten rid of as a mistake. The essence of Creation needs to be allowed to vibrate and evolve so that Form can come into alignment with Loving Essence. Manifestation is the way in which essence experiences itself so that it can evolve. Beginning with yourself, by releasing your limitations so that you can expand into your full self, you can gradually expand your loving acceptance to include all of Creation.

INNER LISTENING

Inner listening is an important step on the path of *Right Use of Will,* but it is difficult and nearly impossible to find in an atmosphere of judgment. Judgments can keep a chatter going in the head, and it can be very critical, not only of others, but of everything you do, including trying to feel more deeply into yourself. Many people are unaware that this chatter is mostly internalized judgments because they have been seeing them as reality. Judgments frame the situation as unable to change. Judgment release is necessary to allow the patterns that judgments have been holding rigid to move and clear the space for inner listening.

Judgments always carry a denial of some sort, and what the judgments have denied is usually seeking acceptance in order to clear itself because it does not feel good to be a denied part of the self. In most people there has been an ongoing conflict between the judgments, or the person's held viewpoint, and the denied truth which has made inner listening impossible without the use of control. Here, meditation that does not exert control can be very helpful for improving inner listening and receptivity. One suggestion is following your breath. Another is to breathe to any place in your Body that is tense or not feeling peaceful. Making sound on the exhalation can be very helpful.

Health is not often achieved in a background of internal clamor that is in conflict about what to do, how to do it, what others will think of it, etc. Habits aren't easily released in this atmosphere either, because the Body's voice can be lost in the ruckus. Most people have been using control when they have not had the idea of listening to everything in themselves as a way of finding inner alignment by ending denials. While inner listening doesn't require meditation, it can definitely help if you are having trouble listening to yourself, or if you think you are listening to yourself, but you have not been finding the depth you want.

Inner listening is a receptive, or yin, aspect. The entire receptive aspect of Creation is needing to be more deeply understood and included as an evolving aspect of Creation. It is not just actions that must evolve; understanding and receptivity must also evolve. The receptive, or yin, aspect of human development has been proceeding with a maximum of imbalance. East and West, yin and yang, masculine and feminine, intuition and thought, feeling and reason, nature and man are still seen as adversaries or as dominant and submissive, superior and inferior by many people.

When polarities are seen as conflicting opposites, and especially when one is favored, the harmony that brings inner balance, and the quiet with which to hear, is obscured by the conflict. Polarities are the evolving limits of One Principle, and so, the answer naturally lies in allowing all of them to come into balance and complementary function. Within each of you are all of these things. The Will needs to be allowed to find balance with the Spirit so that the receptivity of the Will can be valued and accepted as equal to the inspiration of the Spirit. Then, balance in your inner reality can be reflected by your outer reality.

Accepting everything within the self and allowing complementary function can enable you to meet any situation with exactly what is felt to be truly appropriate; nothing more, nothing less. In this way, you are not needing to deny anything; and yet, in trying to allow everything, many people have felt overwhelmed because they had denied something. Without realizing it, they were trying to accept everything outer without first accepting the inner. There were denials of parts of the self tied into misunderstandings about right time and acceptance. The denying consciousness has often attempted to fill in the gap left by denial. Judgments have often served this purpose as people have attempted to make sense of their overwhelm. Denial of the

Will has often been filled in by false feelings that the person has become convinced are real.

Many people have been allowing the media and other people to entirely fill their already clouded receptive centers in an effort to fill an emptiness left by denial. If this source of filling yourself were to be turned off for a while, and you did not find some other way to distract yourself, you might find out how you really feel about the denial of Spirit, Will, Heart and Body on Earth.

Most people, when confronted with this, have tried to fill their mind with thoughts to avoid what they have denied. If you have intent to heal, you need to let yourself feel what you have not wanted to feel, and let it express as sounds. You may feel terribly lonely and afraid underneath everything else. You may have experienced fear of being so ridiculed, or rejected, that you have believed it was the last thing you ever wanted to feel. You may have fear that you cannot vibrate yourself enough to stay alive. You may have beliefs that have told you that fear is a lack of faith in Me; but where am I, and who am I, that I would leave fear outside of My Love? Maybe you are lonely to feel a real presence of My Loving Light there with you. Maybe you are afraid of death, and maybe you are ashamed of your feelings.

Denial of the Will has created an imbalance in the Heart. Unconditional love cannot manifest from this imbalance. The alignment and balancing of polarities aligns and balances everything in-between them. Ending your own Will denials and the accompanying judgmental patterns is going to allow you manifest unconditional love.

This process for ending denials is the only process I have seen to work. The attunement of inner listening is an important, self-empowering part of this process. You can learn to receive input from your own Spirit more and more clearly and, also, to hear directly from Me. Inner listening is one aspect of getting help with the specifics of your own denials. Fear and confusion may come up around this and may need extensive movement because, in addition to your Will, your Heart and Body can also give input here. You may also have internalized a critical voice or voices trying to tell you what to do. You may even experience this as overwhelming confusion, especially at first, and it may be difficult to understand and sort these things out. By persisting with this process, you can find the understandings needed and find increasing trust for expanding the spectrum of your perceptions.

The gift of *Right Use of Will*, here, is that inner listening is easier when all the aspects of your being realize that nourishment from and receptivity to My Loving Light are to benefit all of your being and not just some of it. Then, the alignment needed can be found.

EGO/ SELF

Many have thought that spiritual growth requires death of the ego or the self. This is not true understanding. Death of the ego, or self, is not a necessary part of spiritual growth. Judging against, putting parts of the self aside or not accepting them is denial of the self. There is no problem with ego/self if it sees itself as evolving with the rest of you. This is a part of you, and like all other parts of the self, needs acceptance. Denials and judgments against the ego/self have created afflictions. Without seeing what denial and judgment have created, these afflictions have been thought to be the reality of ego/self.

Ego/self is as divine as anything else. It is the part of you that recognizes you as you, and without it, you cannot tell the difference between yourself and anything else. Ego/self operates to protect your present level of ability to accept, experience and express. Many have judged self-love to be selfish and have had a habit of self-denial as though this is more loving than love of self. To be without ego, or to cultivate selflessness, has often been equated with oneness, but this would be a oneness without differentiation and, thus, no manifestation of Creation. While this has been a goal for some, this is an unrealistic image of Oneness.

As soon as there is a recognition of consciousness, there is differentiation through recognition of the self that noticed this. The awareness of self was blamed as the initial cause of separation. Creation manifests from consciousness. Without recognition of consciousness there is no way to experience it, and thus, no experience or evolution, and ultimately, no existence.

Healing the ego/self with understanding and loving acceptance is another aspect of personal growth. Balance between love of self and love of everything else is what is needed.

FREE WILL IN THE PRESENCE OF OPPOSITION

The question of freeing your Will in an atmosphere that doesn't appear to accept it, is the next issue to be discussed. The question of practicing *Right Use of Will* among people who do not yet accept, or understand, these ideas is a matter of personal choice. It should be understood, however, that there are many obstacles to doing this in an atmosphere of restriction, and that the overpowering of others in any direction, even with ideas, is not the practice of *Right Use of Will*.

Free Will is an old confusion in Creation, which is why so many do not appear to be in acceptance of it. Many have thought that free Will couldn't work because the Spirits were too foolish to make wise choices. Many have feared that they couldn't conduct their own lives well. Many have thought it was not possible because there would never be an alignment. These are some of the reasons that many began to abdicate their own Will in favor of what they thought was My Will.

Many people know that the reality around them is of their own creation and that it is also their reflection, but many have not yet understood how much of their reality has been created by what they have been holding in denial, outside the spectrum of their awareness, and thus, their acceptance. The reflection of non-acceptance for free Will is going to be found to be based in your own misunderstandings, denials and judgments.

Evolution of the individual Will is an important part of spiritual growth, and learning from experience is an important part of evolving the individual Will. Because others are not the cause of the suppression of your own free Will, the practice of *Right Use of Will* does not need to force ideas on anyone or on society at large. The space to practice freeing your Will comes from within you.

Some people may want to seek ways to find others who understand and accept these ideas. Some may want to talk with others about the idea of freeing their Will because they don't want to feel alone in what they are doing. Mutual support can be good. Any lack of receptivity here, is a signal to find these places of judgment and lack of acceptance within yourself. Any seeming conflicts or disagreements can be more easily resolved by finding alignment within yourself first.

If you recover your own lost Will, you will find it much easier to change reality to suit you, than to try and change an outer reflection of denial that you haven't changed within yourself. Finding the balance point between changing the circumstances around you and changing your circumstances is something that each person needs to find, according to how it feels.

If your needs are being denied you by someone else, and you feel you have done all you can to release limits you have been holding on yourself, then you can try changing your approach to fulfilling your needs by finding another place and/or another way in which to fulfill them. Instead of making any judgments here, give freedom a chance to work by allowing yourself to make whatever changes you feel the situation calls for. If this stirs fear in you, try giving it expression as sounds. Remember to make sure you feel safe when you do this. This fear may be holding judgments in place that having ideas different from the mainstream will be ridiculed, censored or viewed as insane, and that you may be outcast or even killed. Having the thought and accepting the fear that there may be repercussions allows you to heed the caution without holding it as a judgment. Freeing your own Will, will enable you to be free.

JUDGMENT RELEASE

Everything is a part of your learning experience. Denial does not open space for improvement because it denies that which could teach it. Denial is held in place with judgments and emotional control. Judgments do not open space for improvement because they substitute criticism and the rigidity of labels for good advice and discernment.

Judgment is not the same thing as discernment. Discernment can draw on past experience, but it also notices the differences. Judgment release is necessary because Spirit and Will cannot find alignment in an energy field locked up by judgments. The inner conflicts that have been keeping attunement away have been misunderstandings, however, if true understanding is to come, full attention to the conflict is necessary. Past experiences are a source of wisdom, but judgments give false wisdom because they do not see the situation for what it really is. Judgments also say that the next experience will be the same as the last experience. This is the same as saying that nothing has been learned, and also that there is nothing to learn that could change things for the better.

Judgments are rigid thought forms attached to the thinker. If you judge your experiences rather than understanding and accepting them, you lock the energy into rigid patterns of perception that take your focus away from what could help you grow. Each time the judgment is made again, and the emotions around it remain unmoved, or intensify, the thought form

17

intensifies. For example, "I'm not a nice person," is a judgment and a label in place of compassion and introspection that could realize why you could have this judgment against yourself.

When negative judgments are held against the self, repetitious experiences will reflect those judgments. Resistance to what is held there can, sooner or later, build up pressure in what is held until it may burst forth as an explosion in which the judgments usually spew forth propelled by denied emotions. This is learning by resisting the lessons until you "meet your match." Reiterating the judgments then, intensifies them, while seeming to prove these judgments to be correct.

Intense judgments are usually made amidst a wave of strong emotion when a person's usual sense of things is overwhelmed, and there is a feeling of needing to push back, "make sense of the situation," or define it. While judgments do label and structure the situation, and therefore, can give a person a sense of making sense of things, they are also limiting. In this way, feelings of not having enough understanding, or personal power, are compensated for by imposing misunderstandings and judgments that bring an illusion of understanding, power and control.

Holding rigid energy patterns that must be broken through by intense experiences is not the only way to learn. Judgments are not necessary steps on the way to understanding. Judgments obscure the ability to use discernment. Discernment in observation and evaluation, learning and experiencing can all take place without judgment. Judgments simplify and rigidify. Judgments are outside of time. They exist after the experience in which they were made, and when the judgments remain, they have the power to influence future experiences to conform to the judgments. This limits your possibilities.

Some people need to release judgments first, before they can accept another possibility or allow their emotions to express. Others need to let their emotions express until they feel ready to release judgments. Don't judge your approach; it may be one way sometimes and another way at other times. Self-acceptance is a necessary component of genuine judgment release.

Heart-felt self-forgiveness has a powerful effect on a person's energy field, but it is also important to use the words that feel right to you at the time. Silent, internal release of held beliefs and judgments is helpful, however, saying the words out loud adds the aspect of manifested vibration. Since this entire Creation is vibration based, actually voicing your release can have a more profound effect than silent release.

Release of judgments helps to free the energy locked up there. Releasing held judgments can be done by saying to yourself, in whatever way appeals to you, that you no longer wish to limit yourself with a particular belief. For example, you could say "I forgive myself for believing…" or "I release the judgment that…" or "I no longer believe that…"

There are many judgments that need release, from the smaller events to the major themes in your life. Some examples are, "I forgive myself for judging and believing for so long that she can never be pleased…that he never listens…that I can never be really free…that anger is destructive."

Releasing judgments in this way sounds so simple, but truly releasing them is not a matter of just saying words. A real shift in how you feel must also take place. There is so much longstanding conditioning that it can take quite some time to shift some of these patterns. Consider, also, the impact of societal habit patterns that speak in pronouncements and, thus, re-enforce the conditioning.

How then to stop judging? Judgment is something you need to feel. Your feelings can tell you when you are making a judgment and, in fact, just feeling judgmental can be enough to create judgments in yourself. True understanding can replace judgments and habitual responses when you can recognize and release the judgments and give free expression to the emotions that have been held there. Then self-forgiveness can come from a place that is real and deeply felt.

In the way that it is the spirit and not just the letter of the law, intent also determines the judgmental quality. If love and acceptance are present, it is possible that statements may have seemingly judgmental words without being an actual judgment. This can include pure humor that doesn't project buried undercurrents. Even so, given that so many people have become conditioned to speak in judgments, it can be very helpful to relearn ways of speaking so that pronouncements are not being made when you say something.

Lost energy, lost love, lost power, lost anything is the result of denial of aspects of the self, of holding them away from you instead of accepting them. What was lost can return when you can forgive yourself for denying it, accept it and understand the possibilities for evolution there. This can mean forgiving yourself for behavior, but more often, it means forgiving yourself for the judgments you placed against yourself for that behavior. You can avoid making further judgments by speaking specifically rather than projecting your present opinions or assessments of a situation into the future with your words, as though this is how it is going to be forever.

The following are some statements that have been believed to be reality, but are actually judgments: "It is a sin to love self; one must love only God. God doesn't talk to people like me. If I think I hear voices, I'll be labeled 'crazy.' No one is going to accept me unless I conform to their expectations. Everyone has to compromise to get along in this world. If I have it my way, I'm being selfish! There's no way out of death or taxes. I have to die of something, so I may as well enjoy myself. There is a certain order to things on Earth, and I can't go against it. The Earth has settled down, so big upheavals are in the past. So many people have prophesied things that haven't happened, that no one can predict the future. God doesn't work miracles on Earth anymore, so maybe He never did. Reality stays pretty much the same. This reality is the way it is, the way it's always been and the way it'll always be."

Judgments are a way of giving conditional acceptance. When the actuality has seemed so overwhelming or unacceptable, people can want to insist that their judgments are the actuality. This is denial of making judgments. However, sometimes people are not ready to face the actuality of certain experiences or the feelings surrounding them. Even though denial has been a survival mechanism at those times, if the intention is for full healing, these denials have to be faced, accepted and understood when the person is able.

Since making judgments stops the situation from changing and sets you up to repeat situations that are held within the framework of your judgments, this has the effect of reducing your perceptions of reality to something that may have seemed more manageable at the time the judgments were made. As I said, these judgments are often forgotten, mistaken for reality and lost into the "subconscious." These situations will, then, repeat until you realize that you are not getting the evolution, change or personal growth that you want in your life.

EMOTIONAL RELEASE

There is another aspect to judgment release, and that is emotional release. Emotion is magnetic energy. Judgments are

20

held in place by unmoving emotions held in the Will. Free Will offers the gift of a much broader spectrum of reality in which feelings are balanced, free flowing, discerning and attuned enough to warn you of any impending harm. In most people, at present, emotions and their accompanying judgments have received many layers of conditioning that you have to accept reality as it is, and also, that deviation is unrealistic, impossible and can have disastrous results.

The Will has been so denied and subjugated that it needs an evolutionary process in order to catch up with present time. When the Will is living in a constricted world of judgments, it is unable to fully surface anything about itself, and so, in the beginning of expressing any aspect of what has been held back, it is going to need to begin in any way that it can. Even though it may look very messy and chaotic along the way, rather than trying to get your Will to comply with a program of release applied by your mind, this is a process that needs to be guided by your Will. The process of freeing the Will from what has been holding it back and what it has been holding back is going to result in finding the needed alignment.

A judgment says that something is such and such, and the more it is repeated, the more it can seem that the judgment is the reality. There are many judgments held directly against freedom of emotional expression. By releasing the judgments you hold against freedom of emotional expression, you help them to show you what they need to express. Being open to allowing whatever needs to happen is part of the process of creating alternatives for yourself, even alternatives that did not exist until you needed them. As you move along in this process, you can reach places of much deeper understanding than you are going to be able to do just by reading about it.

Especially in the beginning, most of your emotional release is something that needs to be done in a private and safe place. If you have fear of hurting others with your emotional expression, it is especially important to move along in this process by yourself until you feel ready to express your emotions in the presence of another. This is because a Will that has been heavily denied is going to be very backed up and may be reactionary and immature when it is first expressing itself. Even so, a Will that is becoming free needs to be allowed to express in its own terms, which at first, may be a lot of words it has wanted to say, but couldn't. These words may contain a number of judgments that need release.

When you give your Will freedom, also do your best not to overstep the boundaries you feel to be present for your own personal safety. Your Will also needs this security. The direct expression of emotions has been so judged against that it can result in intervention of many kinds. As you gain more understanding of what you have been holding in your Will, you will also gain more clarity about what is appropriate in terms of free Will expression in the reality of your daily life.

When people seek to resolve emotions with words or discussion alone, they may think they know what they are feeling when they really don't. Words alone do not give acceptance to the Will's own way of expressing itself. While words can be helpful at the right time, emotions need to be given the freedom to express with sounds. Emotions have a role to fulfill that cannot be denied in favor of the mind or anything else. They may even need to be encouraged to express as sounds that are not managed or controlled by the mind. It is not balance of Spirit and Will to use your mind to tell your emotions how they should be feeling or how they should be expressing. Emotions are not meant to be dismissed or managed in this way.

When emotions have arisen in response to a situation and have not been given complete expression, they do not go away; they subside and wait. Emotions have a presence of their own, and so, when the next situation arises that reminds your emotions of the previous one where they were denied, your emotions may not feel they can respond freely to the situation. The emotional response will be colored by the earlier denials. They may hold back until the pressure builds up to an eruption. These are often efforts of the Will to express not only response to the present situation, but also what has been backed up from previous, similar situations. You may feel this as added pressure from the remaining residue of the unexpressed emotion that has been held back. This old charge, and the judgments made against your emotions' free expression, both need to be released before your emotions can respond to the present situation for what it is.

The usual pattern, however, has been to repeat and increase the earlier denial and put more pressure on the Will if that expression feels like it is going to be more intense than what appears to be appropriate. Instead of allowing free expression to the emotions, this pattern of suppression has been so pervasive that emotions usually only express in situations where they have had some acceptance in the past and in ways that have been accepted. This is why so many women have converted all of their emotions to crying and men have converted theirs to anger.

Instead of having the freedom to be self-determining, the Will, then, is being managed and controlled by outer direction. These are severe limitations on the Will's ability to evolve and integrate. A helpful solution for this problem is to remove yourself from the triggering situation, and allow your emotions freedom of expression in a private place. This will give you a chance to get to know this part of yourself better than you do now.

Sometimes, pent-up emotions, or old charge, build up to the point where they have caused the Will to do things that have seemed to prove the judgments against it. Alcohol and drug use have often provided openings through which judged against parts of the self have found some expression. Then, people have often said it was the alcohol or the drugs and avoided taking responsibility for the pressure they have on their Will.

The emotional body in many people has taken on the appearance of something so dark, alienated and destructive that many spiritual teachers have perceived this to be evidence that the emotions should be controlled or even gotten rid of. However, this would not be the appearance of the emotional body if it were given the acceptance it needs to bring itself into balance. By mistaking judgments for reality, it has long been thought that people must rise above their "lower nature" and abdicate, or let go of, these parts of themselves in favor of their idea of Spirit.

Many people who have said that they want to help increase the spiritual presence on Earth are still holding judgments and unmoved emotions that have been limiting their ability to know what a healthy Spirit on Earth is supposed to be like. Many of these people have treated more feeling-based people as though they are less evolved and have implied as much, or even told this to them. Many therapists, and others, in positions of "authority" have also done this. These people have had confusion about manifestation and what it means.

The magnetic energy is the part of Me that holds manifestation present, but this does not mean that it is supposed to be locked into a Form by judgments. The magnetic energy is an equal part of Me and is not to be judged against or denied. No part of the self is to be denied. The self is not to be viewed as something to shed in order to attain enough enlightenment to reach Me. I want this Creation to evolve, not go back on itself. I want companions.

I want pain, suffering and death to end as soon as possible. Pain, suffering and death are the results of denial.

The Will is meant to guide and protect you. The reason the Will has not been able to do this is because of the denial it has received. To end this denial you need to open into unconditional acceptance of your emotional expression. If you immediately fear, upon reading this, that you and others will get violent and do harm, you need to realize that you have undermined your Will very seriously. In this case, the most helpful beginning point would be to go to a safe place and, without harming yourself or anyone else, express rage with sounds.

Keep doing this until you have expressed enough, and released enough judgments, to be able to trust that you can express your anger without having to control a need to be violent. When you are allowing this emotional expression, do not calm yourself by talking to yourself or force calm in any way that indicates you do not have acceptance for this rage. Calm needs to come from release of rage. This can actually be a good starting place, because the intensity can release a lot of old charge at once. As long as you are in a safe place, you can let this expression take any form it needs to take, including feelings of hatred for others, hatred for your rage and whatever other feelings you have with it, such as powerlessness or feeling unacceptable. When rage is allowed to express, it can often sink into grief at some point.

Intense release needs this understanding: As long as you are in a safe place, loss of control is only bad if you hold judgments against it. Loss of control can actually allow you to break up old habitual patterns of response. Do be aware that extreme rage can sometimes break off from your normal consciousness, making it difficult to remember what you have done. Do your best to stay in that safe place, so that you do not act out. If you have fear about what your rage might do, making the sounds of that fear could help. You can also ask for My Loving Light to be present to protect you. In doing so, you may find out that you are enraged at Me, or at least at the images of Me that you have. Expressing rage at Me is also alright. I have unconditional acceptance for what needs to vibrate in the Will to bring healing.

Now, My Light wants to give some more information on what is meant by emotional release. When you have any feeling of emotion come up, feel it in your Body until you have an urge, or even a nudge, to express it in some way. Then, express in the way your Body is urging you to do. If you cannot make sounds at first, make whatever sound you can, even if it is a little moan or peep. If you need to start with words, let yourself do that. If you do this enough in each situation, you can loosen yourself up and reach what is called ignition. Ignition is the point where your emotions take you over temporarily and do exactly what they need to do. You need not control this in any way other than to make sure you do not really hurt anyone.

Part of this expression may be movements such as thrashing, kicking or rolling. If you feel you must act out in some way, you can use a pillow, or something else, as a symbol of what you want to act out on. You can hit or beat, but bring your awareness present so that you realize you are acting out, and do not do this to another living being. If your emotions want to make sounds, do your best to allow it. It is important to surrender to the expression while it is happening, and let it take its course freely. Be in a state of openness and acceptance as much as possible, and express in this way until you feel no further need to do it. Let your emotional movement show you what it has been holding and what it has to teach.

Pay attention to everything that comes into your consciousness at this time. Other emotions may have some presence there. Let everything that happens find acceptance with you, instead of denial. When the expression, or movement, of your emotional release subsides, rest, drink water and remain open to what else may want to surface in your consciousness. Judgments may surface. If not, seek the judgments you feel ready to release. Threads to other similar incidents may appear. If not, seek the threads, or patterns, that connect this experience to other similar situations. Be open to understandings. This may take many more sessions than you realize when you first begin to contact what you have been holding.

If you do not find love right away for the parts of yourself that have been held outside of your acceptance, you can start by finding compassion for yourself. Looking deeper may be what you need, or you may not be finished with those feelings and viewpoints. You can let more movement happen when you are ready. You can ask for My Loving Light to come into these places.

The understandings you can receive from doing this are not anything I can put in a book. Each of you has your own karmic path to resolve and this process can greatly accelerate it. You may find that your emotions have so much to teach you that you did not realize previously, that you may soon find you want your emotions to surface and release their old charges so that you can open space to receive My Loving Light, gain understandings, remember your past, learn and begin to feel free again. You will find that you feel better, and your Body will feel much better when it no longer has to hold what you have been suppressing.

In some places in your emotional body, you may find some old charge that you fear and/or old charge that has too much fear of rejection to come forth easily in this release process. It is important to trust the progression in which your own Will wants to surface these held charges. The Will has many things layered into it, and this must be respected. The progression you are going to experience is going to be the right progression for you, so do not try to jump ahead to where you think you want to go or pressure your Will, or someone else's Will, to express as you want it to express or to be where you think it should be. Remember to ask for My help, and accept the help I send. I may speak to you and give you some guidance here, or your desire may draw an experience to trigger the movement you need when you are ready.

Although, at first you may feel more confused and frightened than you have ever been because you do not yet know what has been running you, this process is going to increase your ability to receive guidance from both your own Spirit and your Will. If you feel you are not ready, you can remain at a more surface level of understanding, but at least let yourself be aware of this, and be as attentive as you can be to the reflections you need in order to deepen your understanding.

Seeking the depth of understandings you need, must be based in emotional movement. You also need to receive guidance from Me and/or your own Spirit in order to surface and process everything you need to heal. Freeing of your emotions to vibrate is what you need to become better able to receive this guidance. If you start where you are and release everything you can as completely as you can, whenever you feel triggered (and I do not mean that if you cannot give emotional expression to everything, every time that you cannot recover) you can free your emotional body rather quickly, especially relative to how long these patterns have been in place. How long this takes depends upon how much denial you have had in the past. Do find compassion for yourself no matter what your situation.

The Will is meant to receive from the Spirit and trust its guidance, and the Spirit is meant to receive from the Will and trust its response. The more you can clear your emotional body, the more openness you will have with which to receive. This will bring you the guidance you need to clear whatever you are ready to clear. Trust is also as issue here. If you fear being misled, get as much movement into this fear as you can and grant yourself space to learn. As your fear is able to vibrate, you will increase your ability to recognize Me as a loving presence and to be able to discern what does not feel loving.

Even though many people do not, at present, think they really want to hear from Me and would prefer to face their own reflection without knowing it, some do want My help. Those who want My help will receive it in one form or another. If the form presented here feels right to you, try trusting that and find out for yourself what this process has to offer. I can see what is for your own highest good, and it may not always be what you want it to be, but it can bring you the triggers you need to recover your entire self and bring it into loving balance. You can pray and ask for the protection and guidance of My Loving Light. You can also pray and ask for help to notice everything you need for the highest good in your own healing while they are still gentle triggers. However, if you want your emotional release in response to gentle triggers, you must pay attention and not overlook, ignore or judge yourself to be overreacting to mild situations.

Your emotional body cannot evolve if it is limited to old habit patterns of response. This is not a matter of what is presently socially acceptable; this is a matter of seeing that the Will on Earth has become so desperate that it must be allowed to vibrate and receive Loving Light now. Past attempts of the Will to recover without the help of the Spirit have not been successful and have resulted in more denial of the Will and more loss of power in general. *Right Use of Will* is allowing the self to be free.

However rocky its beginnings may look, the balance needed in order to manifest unconditional love will come in the Age unfolding on Earth now. This, however, does not mean that you should abdicate your own participation because you think everything is taken care of. This is a personal imbalance. If you want to participate, you need to find what you have judged against and denied in your own self, and bring it within your own loving acceptance. However, if you are, at first, unable to accept this information, this does not necessarily mean that it is not right time. Allowing your feelings to express and gain the vibration necessary to receive the light of understanding can bring you to the place of right time to end your denials.

As you move along in this process, the attributes of the Will can become more able to balance with the Spirit's overview, inspiration and other qualities so that you know what is pleasant and possible for you in any given moment. This balance in the Heart is what creates a reality that allows needs to be met without overriding anyone or anything.

All the gifts of *Right Use of Will* can come to you when you really align with accepting them by allowing your Will the freedom of expression it needs. You can open space for change by letting your pent-up emotions express as the sounds they want to make and release the accompanying judgments as they surface. This allows the energy to move and vibrate.

REALITIES PRECIPITATING TOWARD EARTH

Opening to the Will's healing and evolution needs immediate attention. The vibrational changes necessary to rebalance Earth are precipitating into physical reality now. Many people are being affected by the physical manifestations of these shifts in ways they do not like because the mental and emotional energy creating these situations has not been cleared enough to allow anything else. The prophecies predicting these times on Earth have described what is going to happen if the understandings needed are not found and implemented. An understanding you need about these shifts is that they do not mean I am judging, threatening or punishing you. What is happening now is a result of denials that have not been able to move in any other way.

Many people have thought that I was a judgmental God. Images of Me as a judgmental God have contributed to seeing Karma as punishment and a balance of payment for sins or debts. Actually, Karma is beliefs or judgments drawing experiences that reflect them. All Karma, then, is essentially with yourself, since what you hold in your own energy field has been drawing your experiences to you. Judgments, Karma, misunderstandings, limitations held on the self and conditioning are all words that can describe the problems of imbalance.

Instead of holding space open for themselves, most people on Earth have been experiencing life as if space were closing in on them, more and more. This appears to you in physical reality as the feeling of less and less freedom in personal life to create what you want, and, instead, a feeling of more and more control, compression and finally death. There has been so much closing-in of space that most people have not let themselves recognize it. Many have wanted someone else to fix it. The fear that the realization would be too frightening and overwhelming has been buried. This avoidance has been allowing the closing-in to progress even more rapidly, because the more the feelings are suppressed, the more unable they are to vibrate space. This increasing compression has been going on for quite some time, and the time has come to reverse this before people no longer have the power to reverse it. Each of you has your own particular amount of spiritual presence and power, and denial has been diminishing it. Inner movement must take place before this power is too compressed to recover its movement and vibrational speed.

Many judgments that control personal reality do not have the final word in world reality. When many people hold judgments collectively, they have a strong effect on the way the larger reality is held. Judgments, however, are not reality and, sooner or later, they trigger their own release.

Emotional release is an important component of shifting the judgments. While I see that the easiest path is to allow yourself maximum response to the slightest triggers until your Will has released enough of its held charge that it can come into present time, I have also seen that so many people have so many judgments against their emotions, are so conditioned away from spontaneous emotional expression, so blocked and disconnected emotionally and so frightened of the pictures their judgments have created about what they have denied, that they have wanted to avoid this path altogether. Many have denied so heavily that they have disowned parts of their Will, and their denials appear to be "others" they have been seeing as the "enemy." In doing this, people are calling for their triggers to come to them from their outer reality. By having this information, you have the opportunity to understand what is happening, to clear as much old charge as possible and to find as much balance as you can. In doing this, you can reduce the intensity of your triggers. In any case, you are not going to experience anything more intense than what it takes to bring your old, buried denials to the surface for healing. In other words, the intensity of your triggers will match the intensity of your denials.

Because emotions have been held back for so long, they have a huge backlog. At first, they can appear to be imbalanced, which they probably are, but given time and acceptance, they will come into alignment. Emotional movement in response to the triggers of your Karma can release old conditioning in the Will, and judgment release can free the mind. You, yourself, can release to change what you do not want to keep the same. If you are thorough in your process, reality will change for you, even if it takes quite some time to shift these patterns. If the judgment patterns are partially released, the energy will start to move, but patterns reminiscent of the judgments will still appear in your life. This is not a curse or a sign that you aren't doing this right. This is to help you see everything involved in these patterns and find the depth of understanding that you need. If continuing to process what this triggers doesn't bring you the shifts that you want and need, you may still be dealing with symptoms and need to seek the cause.

I am guiding this process so that it becomes a successful clearance process for all of the Spirits involved. I am putting everything in its right place so that reflections necessary can be faced without involving anyone other than ones needing that particular reflection. This action on My part has looked like judgment day to the ones foreseeing, but it is only judgment day in the sense that everyone is going to face his/her own reflection. The understanding needed is that this does not mean it cannot be pleasant. Healing yourself in the ways being described here, at the right time and in the right place can release your pain.

The Spirits I have created are not all alike. People's true feelings are meant to guide them to their right place, but denial of the Will has been so extensive that many Spirits cannot find their right place unless I help them. I have many different ways to be and experience Myself, and I do not want limits on any of them. If you have a need for limits, trust that that is right for you at this time, but you must not impose your limits on another. Others have different feelings and different paths, and everyone needs to be free to follow their own path in their own way and with their own sense of timing. Even if you do not understand something; accept its right to be. I want to put all Spirits in the right place for them to grow and learn without the strife that has been going on as different kinds of Spirits vie for the freedom to do as they want to do.

Nothing happens in Creation unless it needs to happen, no matter how it may look to you. Even if most of the Spirits on Earth are having experiences you would not want to have, and even if experiences are happening to others for reasons you do not yet understand, even appearing to be for no good reason at all, you have the opportunity, and can make the choice, to understand why what is happening to you is happening, and release yourself from having to face your denials in outer reality as much as you can. Whatever choice you make will be the right choice for you. Even if it turns out to be a painful choice, you will only experience what you need to experience in order to learn what you need to learn, no matter how much power the reality of others seems to have.

An understanding you need about protecting yourself when you are surrounded by a reality that does not seem to agree with your own personal choices is this: Get in touch with why you are there, process everything you can find in yourself regarding this, in the way that I am explaining here, and see what happens. I am going to help you with this, because I can see that the reality on Earth is pressuring for widespread conformity. You also need to do your part by developing and using your discernment. By taking responsibility for yourself, you can clear up everything that holds you to a reality, or part of a reality, that you do not like. Because misunderstandings have been in place for so long, this can seem to be a tall order; much more complex than many people have thought when they began, but if you do not begin, you cannot get there. When you no longer have anything within you that attracts what you do not want, your right place will feel good to you because it will not have anything that you do not like.

I am not sending any Spirits to what may look like Hell to you unless their denials are so extensive that they refuse to accept anything from Me. What may seem like Hell to you may be Heaven to them. I feel I need to mention this because so many teachings have said that man is base and that, if he gives in to his true feelings, he will bring Hell to Earth or be condemned to Hell.

To bring your own Will into balance, it is necessary to give in to whatever you feel in order to find your true feelings. By giving direct, emotional expression to whatever you feel, you can find your true feelings, which may be hidden underneath your usual spectrum of acceptance. Your true feelings are not in opposition to Me, but you must allow whatever you feel so that the warps and twists on your judged-against feelings can have a chance to evolve. Through this process, they can come into alignment.

I am Love, but confusing self-denial and guilt with love has resulted in many people feeling afraid to make the shifts necessary to end their denials. If people are not ready to accept this information, I will accept their choice, but they will not be able to have this choice on Earth. Earth's time for harboring denial is over. These denials, and the resulting imbalances, have gone as close to the tipping point of being unrecoverable as I can let them go. I want this denial ended now. The pain present in that which is loving, but has been held outside of love, is unbearable and must be healed. Denial has allowed many to ignore this pain for a long time, but I am not disconnected from it. I want you to take responsibility for your own denials.

The Earth can no longer remain hospitable to denial and imbalance, and so, only those Spirits who are in harmony with ending denial and finding alignment and balance are going to be able to remain on Earth. Fear needs to move around this. The fear of displeasing Me is a very great fear on Earth, which also includes those Spirits who blame others and those who have been rebelling and acting out to "show" Me that they don't care what I think.

All the Spirits who originally came to Earth overstepped their limits of right time and right place and experienced things before they were ready, that overwhelmed them and with Spirits they could not accept unconditionally. All of you have been holding fear of displeasing Me in common, even if it presents as anger that says it doesn't care. All of you fell away from Me into experiences for which you were not really ready, and all of you have suffered the consequences. Many Spirits have believed that this was punishment from Me. Many have seen Me as judging or threatening them when I have tried to show them their misunderstandings. Many have tried to push My presence away in the belief that I, then, would not be able to see them or judge them. As painful as many of these experiences have been, they were needed because understanding could not have been gained another way, or it would have been.

I am not judging you for this. I understand why this happened. I seek to help you, and warn you, so you can release yourself from the path of pain and suffering. Many things have been forgotten and lost under the layers of conditioning that have resulted from repeating and repeating re-enactments of old misunderstandings. I have not been sending you pain as punishment. Pain is supposed to warn you that you are going past yourself. Pain only continues if you continue to refuse its messages. However, by overriding or ignoring parts of yourself, many of you have created a long history of denial. Extensive denial has created many situations in which it has seemed that there are no completely pleasing and harmonious possibilities. Life has seemed to be compromise, overlooking things and choosing the lesser of two evils, when, in fact, it could be much more happy and pleasing than that. Beginning wherever you are is the important first step, and finding your true feelings will let you know where you are.

Many Spirits have been having trouble believing in Me, believing what I have said, and that I have said anything lately. I have let this experience go on on Earth for as long as I can. I am speaking, now, to all the Spirits in the form in which they can receive Me, because even the ones who still want to refuse to hear Me, must at least accept from Me the power to put them in their right place. Spirits who are not ready to hear from Me will be put in their right place, where they will not have to hear from Me until they are ready and where they will no longer be mixed in with the ones who want to hear from Me.

Earth has reached the place where her balance must be restored. Those who remain on Earth will have to accept and understand what the Earth needs to be healed. Earth must clear the denials she has received from those who have been living upon her. Earth can no longer tolerate the abuse she has been receiving and, for that matter, neither can the animals.

The animals, for the most part, have appeared to submit to what has been done to them. In their denial of the animals, people have mistaken their patience for lack of response. As people have shut themselves off from most of the animals on Earth, they have lost more than they have realized. Animals have much more to their behavior, and what's more, to their potential, than most people, at present, have been willing to acknowledge, or even notice. Everything needs acceptance and the opportunity to fulfill itself. Animals need the freedom to restore and heal themselves, too. In intense situations, as have been happening now, on Earth, fenced and caged animals need their freedom to have a chance to survive. Domestic animals may need their freedom and the opportunity to return to familiar surroundings. Some animals may become suddenly fierce and unapproachable. Some may choose to die. Cattle, for example, have asked Me to lift most of them off Earth.

Today, many people have been claiming that their knowledge and understanding is greater than ever, but this is not exactly true. While people have more information and experience than they have ever had before, it has all been filtered through the widespread denials so present on Earth and is an elaborate mindset that reinforces mass unconsciousness and the denials that have put this in place. The denials have been so great that people may as well not have had the experience, unless they are going to open to a wider spectrum of awareness, and let it teach them.

So many on Earth overstepped cautions given to them by Me, overloaded themselves and then denied it rather than admit it. In this experience, many Spirits judged against their self-determination and their power. Many lost power, and life on Earth has taken the form of these imbalances and denials. Other Spirits, who had a hunger for power, have attained a place of "power" over others by taking advantage of these denials. Denial of personal power allows others to seem to have more. When responsibility for these denials is not taken, a picture of power can be projected onto others and, then, labeled as causal.

Since most of the ones doing this were not interested in what I had to say initially, they initially set out to prove Me wrong. Denial has caused more and more people to blame others and not take responsibility for themselves. I am not telling you the specifics of this because your own feelings need the opportunity to surface your own memories and your own reasons for being involved. It is up to you to do your part. What you experience as a result of what is happening on Earth is a matter of personal choice. You can find the balance necessary to live in harmony with everything in the way that is right for you. While many people have thought they have this harmony, it has been at the expense of their own Will. Finding the balance in your Heart, by bringing all of yourself within love, is what needs to happen now. This is the survival path.

By seeing and understanding how situations have been created on Earth, you can learn how to shift reality for yourself. You cannot avoid it by denying that it is happening. You must seek the way to create differently. The held fear that you have created your own just punishment by overstepping My guidelines needs expression and judgments forgiven so that, instead of drawing to yourself what you will tend to see as punishment, you can receive My Loving Light. Denying that you have this fear only disconnects the fear from the understandings it needs. Understanding is that all of these experiences were needed for you to learn or you wouldn't have been having them. However, understanding, and understanding the specifics of your own situation, cannot penetrate deeply enough when held fear is blocking the way. It is important to give acceptance to this fear, and let it express itself so that it can both give and receive understandings.

Although the form has been changing, history has been repeating patterns because the understandings needed have not been reached. It has been believed that a change in form would change the outcome, but in fact, consciousness can enlighten or corrupt any form it uses. Many have been denying the reflections of their own denials. These denials will deliver their messages, sooner or later, and the forms this will take will be the forms needed to break through the resistance and oppression they have received.

So, see that the clearing of misunderstandings and the resultant denials is of extreme priority if you do not want to manifest the experiences that will reflect these denials. This information is meant to let you know what has been being held in the mental and emotional energy surrounding Earth. This held energy can precipitate into physical reality, unless those who have created it make changes in their energy fields. You have the choice to recognize this in the mental and emotional levels of vibrations, and shift it from there, before it precipitates into physical reality.

If the denials being presently held in the emotional and mental energy of the Spirits on Earth do precipitate into physical reality without making sufficient shifts in these energies beforehand, it will be seen, and I exaggerate not, as doomsday. However, if you accept your own denied and suppressed lost Will and bring it within love, it can also be seen as the opportunity you need to align your Spirit and your Will in your Heart. The more clearance you choose to do at the mental and emotional levels, the less outer reflection of these imbalances you will have to face.

The wish to maintain denial can perceive the mention of that which is denied as threatening. If you feel threatened, you have a great deal of pressure on your Will; otherwise you can appreciate the warning. These words are not meant to sound like a threat, but if they trigger your emotions, letting them express as much as they want to, can speed up your process.

I am willing to help in whatever way My help can be accepted. At present, the openings through which people will allow help have been very limited by judgments, denials and separations. Help must match the openings to receive it. When emotions are held back, they clog up and block receptivity. Do not underestimate the power of your feelings. If you ask for help while emotions are held in place by the belief that you don't deserve it or cannot have it, this held energy can prevail to the point where help will have to take the form of trying to trigger these denials.

Disconnected feelings can take form in outer reality in many ways. Some Spirits have had a death wish which they deny, and some have believed that they would rather die than face their denials. Both of these patterns have been heavily denying their own denials. Examples of the reflections of these denials are that man has been ravaging, poisoning and destroying the Earth while claiming that life is better than ever, and suffering more ill health than ever, while claiming he is only better diagnosed. Some have been saying that it doesn't matter or that none of this will affect them, while denying the awareness that could notice they are not vibrating enough of themselves for this to actually be true. The threat of nuclear war and the proliferation of radioactivity, while claiming there are no viable alternatives, are the most macabre reflections of these denials. Rather than being given direct expression as emotion, the acting out of anger held in a state of denial, and judged to be destructive, has been building weapons that could destroy the entire Earth, while claiming that these weapons are only to ensure peace and are not to be used.

The practice today of overriding the Earth, the animals and the people with pollution and other death-creating problems over which they have been given no real choice, is not the practice of free Will. However, this could not be happening if the vast majority of people had not already overridden their own Wills. While it is possible that some pollution and poisoning could have taken place as a reflection of the imbalance of Spirit and Will, learning takes place before death results unless the denials are so substantial that death is all they can create. The massive attempt to kill Earth has been being carried out by Spirits who have this much denial. These Spirits have been denying others in favor of themselves. The ones denying themselves in favor of others have been handing them the power to do it.

Once denial is cleared from the Earth, people will find that they really are compatible. Government, if needed at all, can then take the role of open-mindedly observing, investigating thoroughly, giving advice and holding the balance points. At present, life on Earth has been manifesting as much of the pretense and reverse of this as people's denials have allowed.

The question of how to have a society without oppression is the question of Spirit and Will accepting the process of balancing in the Heart. Presently, most people's feelings have been so disconnected from the consciousness that they have drawn experiences without the understandings of why these experiences are happening. When emotions have been relegated to the position of having nothing to teach, and instead viewed as something to control, manipulate or get rid of, events can appear as though random. When people do not take responsibility for all of themselves, the result can often be blaming others and acting out on others. When denial is ended and responsibility taken, balance can be achieved without the extremes of imbalance reflected as injustice, crime, violence, rebellion, war, revolution or any other form of social upheaval.

If you deny yourself past the midpoint, you risk losing the power to keep yourself alive. This is the actual state of many people on Earth right now. Instead of allowing this denial to continue until it precipitates the destruction of Earth, I am intervening. I will not allow Earth to be destroyed by any of the means now being employed because the death-wish of some would override those who want to live; but, I do want to warn you that your own denials could bring these experiences to you. Everyone is going to get their own personal choice, whether they are fully conscious of their choice or not.

Everything being done on Earth right now to try to halt the destruction is necessary, and a part of the process of individuals reclaiming power over their own destiny paths. I want to point out, though, that inner work is extremely important. You don't know what you are really facing "out there" until you find it in yourself. I will help in whatever way is appropriate, but I cannot lift this struggle off of Earth until enough has been learned that these same patterns will not be recreated or drawn back to Earth again. The Earth does not want to be inhabited by those who disrespect her any longer.

Those who have been feeling victimized by the situation on Earth have something to learn here, too. When personal denial is ended, everyone actually does have enough power to protect the self from harm. The end of personal denial allows the Will to create a place for itself that is free of denial and what denial has been creating. Do not hold any limits on the possibilities here.

The Will wants to be freed to find balance and has been attempting to recover through any avenue it feels might be available to it. When the Will has attempted to express as much held emotion, or old charge, as possible in situations that have triggered it, the

Will's attempts here have usually been misunderstood and heavily judged against. A free Will is not destructive as society has feared. When the Will is trapped in a web of judgments, its attempts to release the pressure of repression and denial have often done the things that society has feared. How could it be otherwise when the Will has been so trapped that it has felt desperate? In this light, it can be seen that many have feared facing their own denials, while believing that they fear the Will itself.

The Will can be encouraged to begin with the things closest to it. By finding the space for your Will to freely express its response to everything you experience, you can begin clearing your energy field. Feel everything there. Accept the Will's messages to you without waiting for an outward experience to prove it right. Understand though, that the Will has to be given the time and space to recover its lost vibration and clarity. Even so, it can still provide you with a lot of helpful understandings and information along the way. If the Will is accepted, every experience you have is a learning opportunity to further clarify your energy field and improve your ability to create what you want for yourself. You are not fully filled with My Loving Light, unless you have fully balanced with your Will in your Heart.

While free Will, when attuned, behaves appropriately, there is no place to start other than where you are. The Will must be accepted wherever it is and allowed to express its held charge safely. This will bring the Will into present time. No matter what anyone else chooses to do, you need only make your own personal choice to create your own reality in this way.

The Will seeks understanding and must feel trust in the Spirit to be comfortable in its search. Will and Body can be forced to serve the Spirit, but this is a form of dictatorship and enslavement; exhaustion, unhappiness, dis-ease, aging and death have been the result. The ability to live a long, healthy and happy life comes when the Will and Body are not forced to do what They don't want to do. Many have fears that doing what they want to do will lead to inertia with resulting homelessness and starvation. Others fear they don't know what they want to do or that they cannot survive doing what they want to do, given the ways things are on Earth, now. Some fear this will lead to all manner of degradation. These are all fears that need emotional movement and judgment release. Rather than making sudden changes, which would be a way of going past your fears, you can see these situations as changing and evolving with this process.

Life on Earth is a constant flow in which feelings either remain in balance or they don't. This is the question of balance between Spirit and Will. Once the old charges are released and spontaneity and loving acceptance are found, feelings can accompany and enhance your life like music.

DISCIPLINE, DEATH AND REINCARNATION

Discipline is a point of real confusion among most of the people on Earth today. Most of it is based in beliefs in the need to control situations and others. People have misunderstood, judged and even made laws based on the idea that the nature of man is essentially base and evil and must be disciplined and controlled. This locked-up energy has been slowing the evolution of consciousness drastically.

Discipline is a direct result of undermining the Will. Suffice it to say that an attuned Will is always appropriate. When there is balance in people, there is no need for discipline. Disruptive behavior, or opposition of any sort, is always an attempt by the Will to express what it can no longer hold. Often the origins are older than the person's present age. Lack of understanding about how to handle this has often resulted in discipline. Allowing direct expression as sounds by whoever is triggered by this behavior can help bring understandings so that the disruptive behaviors can be resolved with the loving acceptance they need. The process of aligning your own Will has to show you the true understandings here, because the misunderstandings around the concept of discipline are, at present, so massive, that it is best approached by letting go of preconceived notions and trying out the process of recovering your own freedom of Will.

The Will must be unconditionally accepted by the Spirit to be able to balance with It in the Heart. The Will has been so severely disciplined on Earth that It is extremely confused and, in fact, is very much like an abused child in most people, full of distrust and held emotions. The Will has been damaged to such an extent that death has been the regular result, and nearly everyone has accepted this as the way it is supposed to be. The fact that death is taking place at all indicates a serious, and longstanding, imbalance of the Spirit and the Will. Death and rebirth are only a temporary way to work with this imbalance.

The maximum possible amount of time has been given for Spirits on Earth to work on this imbalance through the pattern of death and rebirth. This has been seen by many to have been such a large amount of time that an assumption has been made that reincarnation is the way it is meant to be. This pattern had its place, but it has also confused many into thinking that they have an unlimited number of lives. This is not the reality of the situation, though, and fear around this has caused nearly as many to go to the opposite extreme and claim there is only one chance. Neither extreme has had the answer, but, in fact, Earth's time has come to end this pattern by finding Heart balance between the Spirit and the Will.

The desire to outgrow things is part of the path of spiritual evolution, but the application of disciplining yourself into actually leaving parts of yourself behind is not accurate understanding. You need to evolve all parts of yourself and not just your higher levels of vibration or the parts you have thought you liked better than your judged-against parts. Evolution is the process through which these parts can change and grow with you.

You came to Earth by slowing down a part of yourself until it became dense enough to be called physical. The process of birth and death came when the power to speed up the dense part was lost in the confusion of experiencing this new vibratory rate. No one allowed the suspicion to surface that this loss of vibratory power had anything to do with suppressing the emotions that were felt there. Most Spirits pretended they were fine and had no problem. Many blamed others for their entrapment. Many have believed that to even be physical was a sin. Death began to be the regular result of misunderstandings, confusions and judgments around physical existence. There are many judgments around this experience that need release. These judgments were attempts to make some sense of a situation overwhelming enough to cause a split between Spirit and Will. These attempts, however, were not true understandings; they were misunderstandings. Release of these thought patterns, and their accompanying emotional charge, will allow the needed understandings to come in their place.

This entrapment caused a breakdown between the Spirit and the Will, and in most people there has been no communication between their Spirit and their Will in this area. In seeking the cause for the entrapment on Earth that resulted in the split between Spirit and Will and the beginning of physical death, many blamed the Will. Many Wills reacted by blaming their Spirit. The feeling of being trapped on Earth, and of the Spirit having to leave Will and Body behind in order to leave Earth, is such an old feeling that many have come to believe that there is no other way. The question of release from this trap is a question of willingness to face the denials that have been going on for so long on Earth. The confusion of consciousness that resulted from the pressure of changing vibratory rates was, in part, a lack of experience. There is no reason to believe that this will always be the case. This is what has been called "the fall." By seeking within and accepting what you find, you can discover your own experience in this entrapment.

This explanation has, so far, been a generalized one because the experience of losing the power to come and go from Earth at will has highly charged emotions around it that need acceptance, expression and understanding. Introduction to its memory needs to be gradual for most people, but you can remember this for yourself by opening your acceptance for these memories and letting them surface as you are ready, rather than deciding ahead of time that such things are impossible, or are only possible for others, as you are an ordinary person with no extraordinary powers.

Memory loss is only an illusion, caused by a held emotional charge blocking the way between you and old memories. Although the doorway to old memories may be blocked by trauma, if you want to remember, and you are ready, you can remember by allowing these held emotions to express even if you can only allow a little at a time. Forgetting has been a coping mechanism to the extent that many have believed that letting go of the past is the right way to proceed. This denial within the self is the reason that the full memory of everything you have experienced is not presently in a recognizable form in your daily consciousness. The practice of *Right Use of Will* can give you the understandings needed to recover the lost power of leaving the physical plane with your entire being rather than with just a part of it.

THE FEMININE PRINCIPLE

Female is the quality associated with the Will, as male is with the Spirit. Feelings have been equated with female and action with male. Just as Spirit is equated with light and a positive charge, the Will is equated with negative, just as female and darkness have been. Women, then, have been equated with negative and negative with undesirable or unwanted. Women have been seen as dark or bad or even as the root of all evil.

In truth, negative is not darkness. The negative charge of the Will is the energy that can vibrate darkness, and thus, open space to receive light. This vibration is the magnetic/emotional energy that can attract light. When it is judged against, it cannot attract Loving Light. People must realize that all emotions, expressing freely within loving acceptance, open them to receive Loving Light.

Feelings, as well as the other aspects of the Will, are a divine and necessary part of every man and woman. It is essential for Earth, at this time, to recognize and align with the negative energy that has been so misunderstood and maligned. When the position of the Will is restored to balance within men and women, inspiration and response will balance and blend according to what is appropriate.

Receptivity and response are meant to be associated with the feminine aspect and inspiration and action with the male aspect in both men and women. The Will is the feminine aspect of My Light and is My Divine Mother Principle.

SEX AND CHILDREN

When children can be born of the balance of the male and female aspects, both within and between the parents, they will also be able to balance and unfold into life on Earth in the kind of family situation that will respect, accept, encourage and nurture this spiritual balance. When children being born can experience an environment that nurtures their true being, the evolutionary process will speed up tremendously. No longer will people have to spend so much of their time trying to recover from what happened to them in the womb, at birth and in the early stages of their life. Children will be able to grow and evolve within the family from the start. It is a real possibility to attune yourself so that any children you have in the future will be attuned to you and to the rest of your family.

Parents, and other family members you already have, may or may not accept this growing spiritual attunement in you. Old conditioning and conditional love has often pressured people so that they have not found their own sense of self, or their own path, very easily. Many have abdicated to images held by family members as to what, and how, they are supposed to be. Family members on Earth, at present, often reflect one another's denials. Some denials reflected by family members are very deep and old. You may be reacting to what you have, consciously or subconsciously, denied and projected there. When this is what's happening, you are not seeing the true essence. This is why it is often not possible to process these denials directly with one another. The complexities of this will unfold as you progress in your process, and is another reason why it is much preferable to process with yourself first. Processing in this way can bring shifts in your relationships with others. Often, finding spiritual balance for yourself can bring spiritual balance to your entire family. This will bring much needed harmony.

Many of the problems on Earth, and within family relationships, can be traced to sex without love or sex with only conditional love. When sex is not given acceptance within My Love, this energy field has an adverse affect, not only on the people involved, but also on the children who may be conceived. When this is the case, the denials involved can manifest in the children, and the accompanying judgments can partially, or fully, block receptivity.

The spiritual sanctity of sex is not in its right place when sex is treated as something dirty, shameful or in other ways that place it outside of My Loving Light. Sex is not meant to be evil, base, lustful, animalistic, or any of the other judgments it has received. Sex is not to be placed outside of My Loving Light by labeling it as something to be outgrown or given up when spiritual awareness is seriously sought. Since the Will has been so denied and misunderstood, the act of physically having sex has often been filled with these denials. Then, instead of a shared loving experience, sexual activity has often been dominated by denials, physical need and a drive for gratification. This creates a separation, or gap, between sex and My Loving Light, in which many things can, and have, manifested that have been very problematic, not only for the people involved, but also for Earth.

The questions that some people have raised about what has been labeled "loose sex" have been founded in feelings that something is not right about it, but it is sex without love, not sex without societal approval, that is what has not been right about it. Instead of each situation being seen for what it is, the judgments have angered many people who have counter-judged that it was just some punitive religious ban and prejudice against people enjoying their bodies. The understanding of the sanctity of sex has been, for the most part, lost, and while understanding was meant to be sought, the presence of these judgments froze the energy field until most people began to think that the judgments against sex were the reality of having sex. This is all going to clear up as people end their own denials.

When people have a sexual relationship, this closeness and focus opens their energy fields, or auras, to one another, and their energy fields mingle together. The love that is present, and also the denials, mingle together. Often, people have not known what is being held in a state of denial there. In sexual relationship, "what is yours" becomes "what is ours." When men ejaculate, they can, and often do, pass denied emotion to their partner. This is problematic, but it is particularly problematic when what is passed is denied hatred of women with a charge of denied rage.

Each person must be responsible to him/herself here, as no one can really be the determiner of this for another. If the ones involved claim they have only love and have not given acceptance to the denied undercurrents they have, they are having sex in the presence of denial. Opening to accepting your own judgments and denied feelings is the most important thing you can do to help this situation. Sex in the presence of denial, and especially sex without love, has been opening space for problematic reflections to manifest and for denial Spirits to enter Earth.

Sexual energy is magnetic. Magnetic energy attracts what it is vibrating to. The love that would naturally connect through sexual closeness is meant to increase Light, Love and Will presence through orgasm, but Will denial is not able to attract Loving Light. Orgasm, with denial in the energy field, has been increasing the presence of denial on Earth. So many people have increased the denial on Earth in this way that the ones able to see it have thought that sex brings darkness to Earth. The true understanding is that sex in the presence of denial has been increasing the darkness on Earth. Not only do the ones doing this increase their own denial and lessen their light, the children they attract to be born through these unions carry the denials that are present between the parents. This has been playing a larger role than most people have realized when these denials manifest in the relationships with their partners and their children, and they dislike so many things about them.

Many people have thought that child-raising was not so pleasant, but was a necessity. Even though most people have been told that it is supposed to be, and claim that it is, a wonderful and loving experience, the truth of the matter is that many parents have been having trouble accepting their own children unconditionally and vice versa. Many parents have mixed feelings about their children, as they do about their partners. Even though many people have tried to tell themselves that this is just the way life is; this is no accident. There is a definite relationship. The more alignment you have within yourself, the more alignment you will attract as a partner and in your children. Wherever there is lack of alignment, you will attract the reflection of those denials. The more lack of acceptance in the parents, the more unacceptable and unaccepting their relationships with their children will be.

Even though most people on Earth have not, yet, experienced unconditional love for one another, this now needs to happen and must not be believed to be impossible. Everyone has had the experience of loving parts of another person and feeling very annoyed, and even hateful, toward other parts of that same person. It has been thought to be that when you love someone, you have to put up with whatever they do that does not please you. This has been called unconditional love. However, what about you and how this really feels to you? When you feel you have to suppress parts of yourself in favor of someone else, this is conditional love that involves self-denial and self-sacrifice that hasn't known how to fully love self and love another at the same time.

An understanding needed now on Earth is that many people, without realizing it, have left themselves open to attract to themselves darkness they have not been prepared to handle. This darkness, then, is in themselves and in their children. It is a reflection of what they haven't accepted in themselves, and it is more than that, too, but is not something that can be fully explained right now. For now, opening to accept your own denials and lack of self-acceptance can greatly improve the situation and help you understand what else needs to happen.

It does not further healing to continue with the misunderstanding that I have asked people to sacrifice themselves for others. Original Cause in Creation had this misunderstanding as a part of it. If you look at this thoroughly and follow it through as many implications as you need to understand it, you will see that it does not work. This includes the raising of children. Children need examples of how to relate in a realistic manner with others and not more examples of how to further deny themselves and others.

In discussing this subject, in fact, it is necessary to point out something else. Any time a parent allows the birth of a child it does not really want, there is an accompanying risk of allowing into the Earth a Spirit who cannot make its own choices well, or even more likely, a Spirit who will override the feelings of others in favor of itself. When Spirits enter Earth against the wishes of the ones bringing it into the world, they often continue the patterns of overriding others. Earth has been reaping the harvest of these practices. In taking responsibility for bringing Spirits to Earth, it is also necessary to realize that the openings made through conditional love have allowed a mixed presence on Earth, and the openings provided without love have allowed loveless Spirits to enter Earth.

Knowing yourself helps you to know whether you really want the child or whether confusion about individual Will and Divine Will is causing you to accept a child you do not really want. In any case, a child not totally wanted is not a child of unconditional love. At present, abortion is actually preferable to increasing the presence of Spirits who will deny others in favor of themselves and preferable to increasing denial in general. Having a baby because others say it is required and abortion is not allowed, brings more Spirits who are not in harmony with respecting others. In pregnancy, both the baby and the mother have to be considered.

If there is an alignment, conception will only take place, no matter what day of the cycle, if the parents both want a child and the right child for them wants to enter at that time. Living with the fear that unwanted pregnancies are a part of life is not necessary. Unwanted pregnancy will not happen if both potential parents are balanced, and also will not happen if you use the method of birth control that you feel is necessary until your Body tells you that it is no longer necessary. If you are on your way toward balance and are making this clear, denial Spirits will not seek to be born through you because they will know that you will not allow it.

During the time that balance is being sought, unconditional acceptance of everything that happens along the way is needed, including any feelings of fear, anger, grief, guilt and loss. If an unwanted pregnancy presents itself, seek the denials involved by looking over everything that presents itself about the situation and learn without making judgments.

The conditioning that sperm are madly swimming for their life toward the egg, no matter what, and that barriers to this are the only hope, need release. Sperm can be guided by the consciousness in which they are ejaculated. This is why some people wanting children and having low probability of producing them are able to do it anyway. This guidance is the consciousness of both potential parents, not just the male. The persons involved must both be clear about whether they want a child at this time or not, and the harmony must be at all levels between them, not just mental or just sexual or just feeling good with one another or any other partial acceptance.

If, on the way to balancing, you are not finding wholly compatible partners, some birth control is still going to be necessary. You can still see the situation as evolving toward a time when the need for birth control is a thing of the past as the balance between Spirits experiencing sex with one another increases the presence of Loving Light, Will and Heart on Earth and guides the process of conception to attract only Spirits in harmony with the Destiny Path of Earth. Rest assured that this can happen quickly, but don't pressure yourself to be there before you really are. Allow yourself the space needed to learn what you need to learn so that you can evolve.

The outer shifts that will bring this evolution are close at hand, and the conception of a child at this time, I want to remind you, is going to reflect your denials as well as your self-acceptance. You will then have a more complex situation in which to find alignment, so, unless you feel you can have unconditional acceptance for whatever is going to happen, I recommend postponing pregnancy. This will not stop anyone from having children later if they so desire. It will protect people from the grief of perhaps being unable to protect themselves and/or their children from the consequences of these denials and from what is happening on Earth. As much as possible, energy is needed now to focus on bringing the self into the balance needed at this time.

You are going to be able to have children, and lovingly care for them with much joy, if you allow yourself to increase your own inner balance first. Having children without finding this balance first can still be a healing path, but may bring more pain for the Spirit and the Will to have to work out. Pain in childbirth, for example, is another expression of less than total attunement between Spirit and Will, and between mother and child. An understanding needed is that judgment here is not helpful. Painful and difficult pregnancy and birth, and also painful child rearing, can heal so that there will be no more painful or traumatic

47

experiences with it. The pain of the Will has increased each time it has given birth without the loving care and acknowledgement of the sacredness of bringing Spirits forth on Earth.

Overpowering doesn't need to happen between parents and children. Children need an opportunity to develop their own responses to situations and learn to choose accordingly. *Right Use of Will* is for all ages. If family is not allowing children to develop their free Will, the children need to realize that they may have chosen this family or there may not have been any other opening through which they could be born. They will have to accept this to whatever degree is necessary and do the best they can to make space for themselves and hold on to their own sense of self until they are able to leave home.

If parents are not intending to interfere with the free Will of their children, but are not sure about what this means, let Me say this: It does not mean letting the children run over you. This would be denying yourself in favor of them. However, do not deny them in favor of yourself either. This is a delicate balance, especially in the learning stages. If the behavior of your children does not make sense to you, as much as you can, discern between your own needs and theirs. For example, you might say, "I understand that you want to do this right now, and maybe you can do it later, but right now, it is necessary for you to do this (whatever it is) with me."

Encourage and support them. Let them learn, and protect them while they are learning. You can give guidance, and let them learn without imposing your reality by requiring them to do, or see, everything your way. Protecting children from danger is necessary, especially in the world at large, but this can be done constructively, without filling them with fear, often by simply being present with them. For example, instead of stopping a child from learning to do things by telling the child he/she is going to get hurt, you could help the child to be successful. Instead of telling a child to be quiet, you could listen to what the child is trying to express. Rather than making judgmental pronouncements, you could help the child to learn. If you feel you need to say something, make your comment specific rather than a generality about the child's abilities.

Trying to keep others where you are is not free Will. If children are seeing things that you do not see, fearing a particular adult, for example, they need to be allowed to have their feelings, be acknowledged and feel heard rather than dismissed or pressured because you see this person as a "nice person. It is important to give acceptance to emotional expression rather than use it to control what is accepted and allowed. If children are angry, see if they can be helped to find healthy ways to give it direct expression other than acting out, and start by giving acceptance to their anger. It can help to express your own anger without frightening the child with it.

Acceptance and acknowledgment can increase children's confidence and self-acceptance. As they grow, they can become more and more able to realize their potential as well as recognize potential dangers or drawbacks. This approach can foster true independence, make the job of parenting easier and create good alignments with the children. Then, when children are ready to leave home they can do so with confidence and balance rather then in reaction to their parents.

If the situation has not been as described here, it can always begin. Starting from where you are is the only point for beginning. You may need to begin by giving expression, privately, to your own emotions. This is often better done in private so that children do not misunderstand or become frightened of their parents' emotions. If you have enough self-acceptance to express your emotions in the presence of your children, this doesn't mean subjecting them to verbal diatribes. It means making the sounds your emotions need to make. Giving acceptance to children's emotions and points of view helps them to communicate and express themselves. Seeing that children and parents are together to learn from one another, and not just the child from the parent, can accelerate the growth. Chances are that time is going to be needed to reach the understandings needed. Allow time to show you what you need to see.

FREE WILL BETWEEN PEOPLE

Mixed presence on Earth has resulted in no one on Earth being able to completely fulfill his/her own Destiny Path. Everyone has been finding they can only do some of the things they want to do. Many have thought that compromise was necessary, but compromise is a judgment, usually in advance of the experience, that the entirety of the proposal is not appropriate or possible. The need for compromise results from denial. Compromise impedes the evolutionary process because no one compromising finds out if their own approach would work or not. Compromise is no more reasonable than denying parts of people in order to force them all onto the same Destiny Path. People can come to agreement freely.

In having believed that free Will carries complications requiring compromise, change here needs to come, and is going to come, as a result of the process of freeing your own Will. This process is going to change relationships and bring many new understandings. No amount of discussion can bring the alignment that freeing the Will can bring. Freeing your Will is going to show you that free Will between people is entirely possible and not in the ways so far attempted on Earth. All of the supposed expressions of "freedom" have involved denials. Denials always involve overriding parts of the self which inevitably leads to overriding of others, either overtly or subtly. The experience itself is needed to learn how it can actually take place that everyone can do exactly as he or she wishes without having to compromise, be overridden by another or be overriding toward another. It will be seen that relating in this way can take place without imbalance or potentially dangerous denials. By starting with yourself, the rest will unfold for you.

The path to free Will is not going to be as easy as it would have been had it been done initially, because there is so much conditioning. So many people have become so conditioned away from the straightforward expression of their true feelings that often feelings emerge sideways or in twisted forms. This conditioning has created a much bigger charge of unexpressed emotions than existed originally. Nonetheless, it can be resolved. Do not judge emotions by what you have seen so far, and do not judge emotions by the ways in which they may need to express in order to recover.

Denial originates with the self and then spreads to others. Because of this, it must be resolved first with the self. These original denials gave rise to more denials, like an advancing cancer. These denials made openings for Spirits who took in these denials to reflect them back to those who had denied them originally. Unfortunately, these denials were not understood according to their origins and were thought to originate in the Spirits reflecting them. Because judgments twist things into the judgment patterns, they can, then, seem to prove that the judgments are the correct interpretation of the reality. Many people had feelings trying to surface in their Wills to tell them that this all originated with them. There were many reactions to this. Some feared they were aggrandizing themselves to feel this way. Some had shame and didn't want to let anyone know what was really happening with them. Others decided to move away from those having trouble as though they were somehow better, and so, didn't have these troubles. This increased shame and lack of self-acceptance in some, while others felt secretly superior and arrogant without realizing it was parts of their own Will becoming lost and isolated in these separations. These misunderstandings amplified until, now, you have the situations that you have on Earth.

The ways of living on Earth, in reflecting these denials, have not been allowing much direct approach to problem solving. There has been a general lack of honesty because so many have been so busy hiding things, but I can see how their emotional bodies look, and it is not a pretty sight. The direct approach could solve the problems that these denials have been trying to avoid, but there has been such a large build-up of distrust and held emotions, especially blame, that many have not been wanting to take responsibility. Instead, denial has been saying that conflict on Earth is supposed to be solved according to laws and procedures that have, themselves, become riddled with denial and arranged to block direct approach. Whether they are applicable or not, procedures are in place. If people don't fit the form, they are supposed to make themselves fit the form.

This is backwards. Form is supposed to fit the people and the situation, but when denials are involved, it also reflects the denials. Some have tried to deny the reflection here by belittling the importance of Form, and others by aggrandizing it. When you have already denied things within yourself it can be very difficult to notice when you are denying others. When denials have reached the point where they seem to be more powerful than the self that originally made the denials, this could be called intimidating form.

Real help is what people need when there is conflict, not a settlement that is enforced whether people have agreement or not. That which cannot align with the settlement is forced to be held undercurrent. Possibilities for denial are increased in this way and so is the explosive possibility of society when undercurrents can no longer be held. Settlement needs to feel right to all parties involved; however, unless there is movement in the Will, there can be no real settlement. The guideline here is that no one has the right to force anything on another.

51

While in the process of clearing your denials, you can aid your interpersonal relationships by observing this simple guideline: Do not impose your approach on others, and do not let others impose their approach on you. As you try this out, you can find out how difficult this can be for you, which will let you know how much guilt you have and what judgments you may have held against taking care of self. You need to look deeply into this to see how much has already been denied in situations of relating to other people. To understand your denials here you need to let yourself feel the actual feelings that you have, and let yourself hear all the thoughts you might normally ignore or try to push away.

As you gain information in this way, you can respond to your own needs and also create freedom for other people to state their needs. In allowing yourself to meet your own needs, try to get to the bottom of them by seeking the source of the needs rather than staying at the symptomatic level. You can seek the source by asking yourself why you have a certain need. If your answer is another need, ask yourself why you have that need. You can follow yourself back this way until you find the initial source of the need and what lack has left you feeling unable to meet the need. If your answer is that you don't know, stay open to further understandings coming later. Denials leave the self feeling incomplete. This is why trying to meet your needs might still leave you feeling unfulfilled. Nonetheless, meeting your needs is still an important step in healing yourself, not only to help you understand why you have the needs, but also for increasing self-acceptance and self-love. If meeting your needs involves other people, the balance point of free Will is maintained when nothing takes place that is against the free Will of another.

For example, you do not need to let other people tell you how you should be relating to them. Instead, you can let that person express his or her feelings toward you, and let yourself feel whatever you feel in response to that. This can provide a lot of information about how you have been relating to others. Rather than trying to get the other person to adjust their feelings, work with your own feelings, and see where this takes you. Allowing the movement of expression of your feelings often brings shifts, either in the way you relate to that person or the decision to stop trying to relate to that person. Seek the judgments involved and release what you can of them. If you decide to end a relationship with someone, try to end it without judging yourself or the other person. Your emotions are for you to feel and express, not for the purpose of judging, coercing or manipulating others.

In seeking balance in the ways being described here, the obstacles can seem formidable. The amount of denial and backed-up emotions can make a direct approach between people attempting to resolve conflicts seem impossible, and sometimes, it is. When backed-up emotions have poured out, labels have been applied by people who lack understanding and by people who are in a heavy state of denial themselves. However, people can recover if they can find ways to express themselves as they need to.

Do not make an assumption that violence would necessarily be involved here. An understanding you need is that repression of the Will's expression can result in violence. Violence is the last resort of repressed Will. Some Spirits have denied their own Wills so extensively that any additional denial by other people can cause them to erupt in violence. You can protect yourself from this by realizing what is happening in your relationships with others. As you notice denial in yourself, you can more easily notice it in others.

You cannot deny yourself without denying others. For example, if you deny yourself in order to do something for another, how is that other person likely to feel if you are doing something for them that you do not really want to do? It either does not feel good or there is denial of how it feels. If you really do want to do something for another, do not claim you are doing it just for them. Undercurrent here is the judgment that the one denying self in favor of another is in the spiritually superior position. Attempting to balance this later by allowing others to sacrifice themselves for you is not appropriate either. Feeling this is what will let you know that My Light is right here.

Time is short on Earth for ending denials, but intent can help open space for you to make these shifts. Even though I have already seen who is ready to make the shifts now necessary on Earth, if you have sincere intent to heal, I still want you to make an open declaration of your intent from your Heart to My Loving Light.

The fact of the matter is that the coming changes on Earth are not going to be easy for many. Many people are going to be lifted off Earth. Many of you need to stay present because you need to experience these changes and learn from them. The recovery of your own true feelings is your survival path. Allow yourself to express any fear, anger and grief you have concerning Me, so these places in you can also know that I am a loving God and be able to receive My Light. Instead of judging Me, accept Me as the kind of Creator who cares about what He has created and accept that My Loving Light is willing to help you. Tell Me, out loud, what your intent is currently and communicate with Me frequently. Whenever you are moving your emotions and/or recognizing and releasing judgments, ask My Loving Light to come into these places where you held yourself apart from Me before. Ask for My help as often as you need to, but do not expect Me to do it for you because you need to take responsibility for yourself now.

THE INFLUENCE AWAY FROM FREE WILL

Long ago, before there was any experience on Earth, the Will was denied in the heavens by Spirit energy that did not understand itself well enough to accept Will energy. The Spirit energy saw the Will as holding it back. The Spirits who manifested this viewpoint wanted to have more expansive experiences than the Will seemed able to accept. The Spirit energy perceived the Will to be in apparent opposition to this. They saw themselves as though they were birds chained to their perch by their Wills. Overpowering of the Will took place in every way it could take place, including disconnect from the Spirit. This split has been in place ever since.

Many times the Will has almost recovered on Earth, and as many times, this recovery has been undermined by something still held in denial. Because the denial was not recognized, it drew, each time, an outward reflection that seemed to deny free Will by stopping the recovery. If this outward reflection had been recognized for what it was, the Will could have recovered. The understandings needed were not there, then, or recovery would have taken place. The Will is not wanting this to happen again. The failure, so far, to entirely recover lost Will should not be judged as evidence that this cannot be done or should not be done because free Will does not work. Free Will needs complete acceptance, and not conditional acceptance, so that it can give its full contribution.

Many Spirits have tried to deny the validity of free Will by saying that it is unwise to grant freedom in advance of wisdom. The question, then, is, how are you to gain your own wisdom without experience?

These Spirits have promoted rules and regulations, procedures and the form of learning from teachers, or experts, who are supposed to know best. Progressing through this form in accordance with approval granted by those controlling the form has had the effect of keeping things repetitively the same. Freedom, which often meant privilege, was supposedly granted in accordance with the candidates' readiness to accept it wisely.

One of the problems with this approach is that someone, or ones, must be set up as judge of what is wisdom and what is appropriate learning procedure for another. While some places have had more "fairness" than others, wisdom for one may not be wisdom for another. Limits for one, may or may not be limits for another. The path of one, may or may not be the path of another. This has been a continuance of the path of original misunderstandings that have denied Me, while claiming authority from Me to continue this denial of free Will.

Many who have accepted the influence away from free Will have also said that doing what you want to do is selfish and even dangerous. This is ridiculous if you really think about it. A judgment held here is that telling others what to do is not selfish, but is, instead, appropriate and for the "good of all." Because of what was judged to be the Will's original mistakes, the judgments have been perpetuated ever since. This is self-denial. You have been given what you need to evolve and fulfill yourself, which is your Will, if you accept it. What feels best all around is to do for others what you really want to do and nothing more. However, given that so many people have guilt and self-denial mixed in with love, it is likely that you will need the practice of *Right Use of Will* in order to be able to live in this way.

DENIALS SHARED BY MANY

There are many judgments that large groups of people hold in common, and so, they also share the resultant denials. I am only going to mention ones that could easily be overlooked because they happened so long ago and because people have come to take them as reality.

All of manifested experience, so far, has been in search of self-acceptance. Attuning the Will is not something that can be left out here. Self-acceptance must include acceptance that individual consciousness emerged to evolve essence. Since I am multi-faceted, there are many manifestations exploring these many perspectives. Finding free Will can show you how these aspects all fit together. Because there has been so much discord, this may seem impossible, but it is not. Even though many have become disheartened, and even hopeless, about this ever coming to the promised Golden Age, it can and it will.

Emergence into individual consciousness is not completed when you accept that you have emerged. Each of you emerged to fulfill your Destiny Path. Self-acceptance must come first, so that you can do what you came forth to do. I am much more complex than anyone on Earth has yet realized. Some Spirits have had so much fear of these realizations, and the responsibilities involved, that they have tried to avoid them by denying Manifestation and Form. These people have believed that having a Body was a sin. However, even though a full alignment between Spirit and Form has not yet been found, Body is the Fourth Part of Me, and can also be referred to as Manifestation. The full self has Spirit, Will, Heart and Body.

Some Spirits have tried to cope with the vastness of My complexities by slowing themselves down and experiencing at a slower speed. Their overload wanted to take things at a speed they thought they could handle. Many of these Spirits came to Earth long ago without realizing how far they had fallen in vibratory rate or that they would be unable to speed up again and leave Earth with all of themselves. Most of them denied that they were trapped here and began the pattern of breaking off from whatever parts of themselves they blamed for their problems. This is how death began and what led to the inevitable need for birth, since no one can permanently abandon parts of the self. Some of these Spirits took the form of animals. When they experienced entrapment there, they often became confused between themselves and the forms they had taken on. Many coped with this by denying their feelings and abandoning the parts of themselves that were trapped. This lack of self-acceptance got stuck in blame and loss of consciousness. The myths about Centaurs, Satyrs, Minotaurs and all other stories about animals turning into humans, and vice-versa, are stories about these experiences.

When other Spirits saw this happening, some tried to help. Denial that these experiences ever took place has greatly impeded recovery here. Reclaiming the consciousness lost there has been a long process, during which most of the ones who tried to help have also become trapped on Earth. The reasons for the entrapment were many and differed with individual Spirits. Many Spirits saw Me as an all-seeing and judgmental eye. Some of them became trapped in animal forms when they sought to reduce their consciousness and hide, or get away, from Me. Others were entrapped by their feelings of not being able to accept the form they already had. Some became trapped in their confusions about limits. Some wanted to experience what they saw as the bestiality of animals. Some feared they were bestial if they were interested in sex. Others became trapped because they thought they had to do what their friends were doing. Still others thought they could learn by experiencing what these trapped Spirits were experiencing. There were many reasons that this experience took place.

This experience was very painful and difficult for those who didn't enjoy the limitations of the forms in which they were trapped. Many judgments were made around these experiences. Many of the Spirits who did not get trapped, judged themselves superior to those who were trapped. Many of them also judged that those who were trapped in animal forms had base and insatiable appetites that drew them to become so animalistic. Many of those who were trapped, judged, in various ways, those who were not trapped and also themselves and others who were trapped. There is a long list of judgments here. For example, "We're incapable of change."

As with judgments, these judgments did not see each particular situation for what it was. The Spirits judging made assumptions based on what they comprehended when the judgments were being made. These judgments were often made in states of intense emotions. The Spirits who lost consciousness without meaning to, have a highly emotional charge around this experience that includes overwhelming shame, panic, terror and rage. Because the Spirits experiencing these emotions felt like they never wanted to have to feel these feelings again, these emotions have still been holding these judgments in place and, consciously or subconsciously, have impacted every reminding situation.

These misunderstandings compounded the problems and made release from the limitations of these forms much more difficult than it would have been, otherwise. Understanding and compassion needs to come in the place of these long-held judgments. Some Spirits do not want life in human form and need to be allowed this experience. Others have lost consciousness from this experience that they really do want to recover. Everyone on Earth has involvement in this experience, whether directly trapped or not, and the emotional charge here has not, yet, been released.

Your healing can be helped by remembering your own past, relative to this situation. You can connect to these memories by being open to anything that tries to surface in your consciousness around this issue. By going into the emotions surrounding what tries to surface, you can increase your awareness. When I showed some Spirits on Earth how to liberate the trapped ones, they had varying degrees of success in liberating the entire consciousness of the Spirits involved. The Spirits involved often resorted to denial of the part of themselves that was so overwhelmed and released the rest of themselves from their entrapment. This experience is another aspect of why most people on Earth, now, do not have their full self present with them.

The Spirits liberated from these animal forms, at that time, were given human form in which to evolve back to their full consciousness. All the Spirits liberated were given human forms whether they were human types of Spirits or not. The main reason for this was that most of the Spirits involved believed their lack of self-acceptance and lack of acceptance of one another was largely due to how different they were from one another. I gave the human form, and the necessary time in which to inhabit it, so that the necessary experience could be gained to learn otherwise.

Many Spirits who have embraced expansive consciousness have held a judgment for a long time that everyone should, and must, have this sort of consciousness the way they do. An understanding is needed here, and this understanding is one of the main points of denial responsible for undermining the recovery of lost Will. Not all of My Spirits are alike, and not all of My Spirits seek the same thing. Some of My Spirits seek reduction in consciousness, compression and death, and they must be allowed to have it. Many Spirits have, so far, been unable to believe that this could possibly be true.

In holding a judgment, the Spirits who embrace life have been unable to see and accept these Spirits for what they are. They have continued to hold the belief that these Spirits really are like them or will evolve to be like them. The judgment that everything is similar in essence, no matter what its form, was a lack of understanding based in feelings of not being able to accept that these Spirits were what they were showing themselves to be. Denial of these feelings led to more denials, such as an attempt to simplify Me and fit Me within their limits. While I see that these Spirits have needed more experience to be able to accept Me on this, I also see that they held undercurrent feelings that they knew better than Me and were going to show Me that these Spirits could change. This was also a denial of the alignment of form and essence. These Spirits have been creating death all around them, and expansive Spirits have been denying this and trying to take them off their Destiny Path in My Name and in the name of My Love. This is not accepting these Spirits for what they are and for what they need.

Denial of expansion has been increasing since it originated, and yet, these denials have been representing themselves as expansion. This is, however, expansion of compression and denial. The form these things have been taking is the outer shape of the inner essence. The problem has been that these two realities, that of loving essence that seeks expansion of love, light and life and that which denies loving essence and seeks compression and death should not be mixed together. It has been because this lesson needed to be learned. That time is over. Right place is going to sort this out now. The experience necessary to be able to accept this from Me has taken place on Earth. Death is unconditional denial of Me. It belongs outside of Me, and has a place you will understand as you are able. An understanding of unconditional acceptance is also needed here. For now, you need only accept this reality's right to be. This does not mean that you are to accept this reality into yourself and embrace death and denial in any form unless you truly do not want life.

The Will is meant to guide you to your right place and will do so if allowed to. This is the way in which you can have the freedom to have experience without destroying yourself. Do not think of this as mostly an outer reality. The Spirits who fell to Earth have been mixed in with this essence that denies life, not only outwardly, but also, within themselves. Recovery of free Will on Earth has been stopped each time by lack of understanding about how to sort this out and by not understanding the need to do it. The time has come to open to Me here, let yourself learn to feel this denial for what is, and let it go. More understanding is needed, and this process can bring it to you as you are ready. This denial of My Loving Light cannot leave on its own. It needs My help to go to its right place. These denial Spirits have been trying to kill loving essence because they have to get away from it somehow, and because of the confusions I have been describing here, loving essence has not been letting it go. This situation cannot change for you until you accept it for what it is.

An understanding needed here is that the difference between loving essence that has been denied and the denial of loving essence, is that the one seeks love, light and life and has been mistakenly denied, and the other seeks to escape love, light and life and has been mistakenly pressured to accept it. This has been further confused by the fact that unconditional denial denies everything, including the fact that it does not want love, light or life. Denial that does not want love, light or life can be felt by the Will, but the Will needs to be allowed to tell you the difference here, instead of being judged against as unloving itself for trying to bring awareness of this. The recovery of your lost Will is going to be able to give you this information, because the original undermining of the Will was involved with this confusion.

The Will has been able to feel unlovingness from the beginning, but has felt extremely guilty about these feelings. Much of the personal denial took place in an effort to prove to Me, and to yourselves, that the Will was not right here and that everyone really did have loving essence. Time was needed for experience to develop discernment and understanding, but without the Will's participation, this never happens. Denial must be seen for what it is. Loving Spirits need to recognize unlovingness and end personal denial of loving essence.

The judgments here were many. You need to find the ones you are holding yourself, but, I will mention some of them. Everyone judged that their kind of consciousness was the best, and many judged that their kind of consciousness was best for everyone. Many Spirits judged that if they were loving enough themselves, they could teach others to be loving like they were. Many judged that I was not unconditionally loving when I told them they were making a mistake here. Undercurrent here was a judgment that they were more loving than I was. Another judgment many Spirits made here was that, in time, these unloving Spirits would come around, that they were just slow. Another judgment made here was that every Spirit was supposed to return to Me, so the ones heading away from Me were going in the wrong direction. The only other judgment I want to bring forward now, as a general judgment that was made by everyone involved here, is that all of you judged against the Will for feeling like it wanted these death-creating Spirits outside of My Creation. Reality is that this is what they seek, want and need. To free yourself of involvement here, you need to recover whatever lost Will you gave to these Spirits in an effort to help them become loving and whatever else you denied there.

Death does not feel at all good to the Spirits who seek life, and yet, you all embraced it and tried to make yourselves accept it. The understanding you need now is that all denial that is not seeking life must go outside of Me. You must separate this reality out of yourself, and let it find its right place by learning to discern between denied loving essence and unlovingness, and unconditionally releasing everything that creates death, be it ever so slight an involvement. You need to do this in a way that denies nothing at all in yourself, at the time that is right for you and in the way that feels right to you. In other words, separating death out of your energy field needs to feel good and not like more self-denial.

Even if these understandings seem overwhelming to you at first, they will become clear in time. Release of these deep denials is not an easy thing to do, and yet, it must be done. The realities needed to show these denials for what they are have been intensifying on Earth, and letting your Will respond emotionally to what is happening can help you recognize and clear your own denials if you let it. Death is not meant to prevail in My Creation, and yes, I am everything and everywhere, even though you may not fully understand what I am saying here.

Originally, many created Spirits tried to force themselves to experience every place because I did, whether they were desirous of it or not. Although the reality of these denial Spirits felt terrible to the Spirits of loving essence, and they had to use force on themselves to experience it, they judged against their own Wills by saying that it was not the reality of these denial Spirits that was terrible for them, but that their own Wills were terrible for feeling this way. When the Will was reacting emotionally to these denials, many Spirits who thought the Will was in opposition to the Spirit, thought that the Will itself was this denial. Many also judged that their Wills were actually drawing, or creating, the death that they were taking in from these denial Spirits. They made their Wills hold this, because they wouldn't accept or allow the emotional expression needed to release it.

The Will of a loving Spirit does not create death. If it is experiencing death, it has taken this in through denial, in some form or another, and must reverse this in itself to escape death.

TWISTS AND TURNS ON JUDGMENTS

Many people make judgments without realizing it. These judgments may be thought to be the answer, or the truth, for that person, but these judgments twist the truth. Sometimes the truth is twisted because the people involved don't understand the truth, don't like the truth, are ashamed of the truth or misrepresent the truth without realizing it. Sometimes the truth is twisted because the ones doing this have intent to twist the truth. Many people have claimed I was judging when they, themselves, were doing it and, in this way, have twisted the truth.

The way to understand the difference between a judgment and the truth is this: The Will must feel the truth for you. There is no way I can, or want to, delineate for you the truth of every situation you might ever meet. Instead, you have been given your own Will, and your Will is going to evolve if you accept it. The Will is meant to feel the situation and give these feelings to the Spirit. The Spirit is not meant to dismiss these feelings or pressure the Will in any way to rearrange these feelings to please the Spirit. The Spirit is meant to accept these feelings and seek to understand why the Will feels the way it feels.

When the Will appears to judge with feelings that seem inappropriate to the Spirit, it is important to consider that the Will may be right, and the Spirit is reluctant to accept this from the Will. If your feelings have been told not to respond according to the way they naturally would, but to respond according to the ways the Spirit will accept, your feelings are clouded with judgments. In these cases, you may not be getting an appropriate or accurate response from your Will until it has had an opportunity to clear what it has been holding here. When judgments are being held and the Will is being allowed only conditional expression, the true feelings are not accepted. A false "Will" is, then, created and accepted in place of the true Will according to what the Spirit wants to be feeling. When true feelings are not accepted, the truth cannot be determined because the Will is being pressured to give false information.

Twists and turns on judgments are extensive on Earth at present, even to the point of claiming that no judgments are being made. However, nearly everyone is holding judgments. In both indigenous and technologically-oriented societies, belief systems have judgments imbedded in them. Many judgments have appeared to stand as truth because they have been removed from their context so that important pieces of information are missing. These beliefs, or judgments, have been presented as though they are the voice of authority that has the right answers. I want to point out here that if the answer is right, it can be felt to be right without manipulation, pressure, coercion, force or threat of punishment to gain acceptance. The truth has enough presence to be recognized by those who have intention to find the truth. However, people's unmoved fear can be manipulated to accept statements as truth when they are not. Those who have not recognized something that others feel is the truth need to be free to seek the truth in their own way.

For many of you, what I am mentioning here is a mixture of what you have recognized for yourself and what you have not yet recognized. I want you to see what they all share in common, and I want you to be able to recognize this thread in other situations. The common thread is death-seeking denial and the denial of being death-seeking denial. Loving essence mistakenly denied seeks acceptance. Even so, the denials cannot be approached directly. Death-seeking denial unconditionally denies even that it is seeking the death that results from total denial. When this kind of denial is encountered in other people, the safest path is to remove yourself. To sort this out, express whatever emotions have been triggered and see if this is a reflection of denials you have made that want acceptance, or not. In any case, processing this with yourself is advisable. As with anything else, death-seeking denial must be allowed to experience itself, but this does not mean that it must be allowed to be a part of you or your personal experience.

Form needs to be mentioned here, also, because form has been misleading people. Denial can take many forms. Some forms have even imposed themselves on people and forced acceptance. Some of these forms know the truth, but have had intent to twist it for their own power gain. Some of these forms know the truth well enough to know that they should not appear to pressure and have become very covert and subtle. Recovering your Will is going to show you all of this clearly. You need to accept the feelings you have, and explore them, so that you can trust them to show you what you have not accepted from them earlier. The examples given here are intended to help you see the form these denials have been taking on Earth, but these examples are, by no means, all of them.

Many have been promoting beliefs, or judgments, to obscure what they have really been doing. In the presentations being made here, there has not been intent to find, accept or reveal the truth. Many twists and turns have been presented to people about education, health, medicine, nutrition, diet, exercise, agriculture, politics, international relations, interpersonal relationships, birth, death, taxes, the legal system, governments, law enforcement, My Loving Presence and nearly everything else. Many judgments are also fed to children in school, as though they are the truth.

The legal system has repeatedly stated that it wants only the facts and has routinely accepted twists and turns on judgments in place of the facts. So far, whenever the legal system has been involved, it has almost always involved an overriding of free Will in the way the "facts" are presented and the settlements reached. Many people feel they have been forced into compliance by a system that has not told them they have any other option or provided them with one. Imposing the same rules, regulations and limits on everyone has been called fairness, but lacks the flexibility and sensitivity to individual needs and differences that an attuned Will could provide.

It is, also, not appropriate for one set of limits to cover entire areas so that people have no place to freely express themselves. Every minority, even if the minority is only one person, has to have a place in which it can freely express itself. Trapping people within society's limits when people have deliberately removed themselves in an effort to escape these limits, and following people out into the countryside to impose limits on them, which, if appropriate at all, would only be appropriate in concentrated population centers, is not the practice of free Will. Even though you can probably immediately think of examples where it seems that this couldn't be the right understanding, intervening is only appropriate to preserve the balance point of not allowing anyone to override another, for example, harming them. When people are trying to get free, they must be allowed to get free.

Another prominent form of denial is the media. The media has been interpreting reality by what it omits and what it includes. Not reporting some things has been focusing the public on a reality that has been selected for it. Even in what has been reported, many of the relevant aspects have been omitted. This has been done consciously in many cases and, also, unconsciously when the ones doing this have held the same narrow view of reality being presented in their reporting. This is a twist on judgments because this information is usually presented as an open-minded report on what is happening in the world. The repetitious presentation of this reality has been programming people to expect things to be a certain way, to remain a certain way and to change according to the ways that have been projected. Presenting information as though it is open-minded, while denying the holding of beliefs and judgments that limit that openness, misleads people.

Advertising also has responsibility here because advertising has been making it appear that facts and truth are being presented while omitting information and grossly misrepresenting the true situation. Even when "facts" have been presented, advertising has twisted them in ways that have caused many people to overlook other relevant aspects. When given their full context, many of these so-called "facts" can be seen to be irrelevant or even lies. Advertising and the media have used many devious and subtle methods to promote the reality they have wanted to project, including seeking to manipulate people by gaining access to their "subconscious" without the people, themselves, recognizing that this is happening.

Many people have seen this, or partially seen this, but few have realized the full implication to the Will. The reality of young children is especially vulnerable to influence before they have the awareness to understand or discern among these influences. Many young children have been very manipulated by the media even as to what emotions they feel. Young children have the ability to feel these things, however, and this ability should be recognized, and encouraged, rather than denied or overlooked. When young children have been manipulated before they have found themselves, they can have a very difficult time finding their true self later. It can also be seen that television has such a strong grip on so many children because they do not have enough of any other engaging reality in their lives to counter this strong influence. Children's television programs, the advertising aimed at them and even the educational programs, all have twists and turns on judgments programming responses and "reality" into children. The bright, glowing colors of the television screen remind many children of the way colors look in other planes of existence that they still remember, and so, these bright colors attract them. It is known that children's minds open and receive the quick succession of projected images without having time to do anything other than take them in. A programmed reality is being presented to them in this way, and this reality is telling them how the world is and how to respond before they have the experience to know for themselves or can find their own responses.

All of this amounts to presenting a judgmental picture of reality on a wave of strong impressions that this is the reality of the world, the way the world works, how the world has always been and how it is going to continue to be. This undermines children's creative imagination, which is how they create their reality, and which is meant to evolve and remain an active part of them as adults. Watching large amounts of media-produced programming manipulates and impairs the development of a child's emotions and has been sidetracking the energy field of many people on Earth. Instead of projecting their own reality, many people have been helping to hold the patterns in place that have been given out by a few people. These few people have, thus, used the media to project and protect a continuance of their own version of reality and have done this while denying they are doing it.

Many parents do this same thing to their own children without realizing it. The creative imagination of childhood is meant to be given freedom and encouragement to develop. Children are not meant to have a programmed reality conditioned into their being. Children are meant to contact the world in their own way, with the freedom to accept what feels good to them and turn away from that which they do not like.

Each Spirit, when it incarnates on the Earth, is meant to be given another chance to gain the understandings needed. *Right Use of Will* can enable the gaining of needed understandings in these areas. Clearing the energy field can open the way for reality to be created according to Heart's desire. If this, in fact, were happening, reality on Earth would be much more fun, have more variety and many more possibilities open to individuals and even many more levels of reality available to those who felt attracted to them. The grip of mass programming has severely reduced this evolutionary process to a very limited and linear progression of near sameness for every Spirit incarnating, especially in the United States and for those following her lead.

Government has also participated in this. One of the ways to pressure for conformity is the passing of laws that force participation in mass consciousness and impede the freedom to experiment with other ways of living. Governments have revealed intent by choosing to enforce or overlook their own laws according to the situation and the influence it will have on their system. It has been to the benefit of those in power to have people programmed in such a way that they believe their personal power and strength are not enough to overcome the oppression. Instead of oppressing, government is meant to study, advise and hold the balance points in order to provide an atmosphere of the most balanced personal freedom.

Intent is needing mention here. This is not a simplistic Creation. Intent to understand Me will guide you to understand Me, and intent to deny Me will lead you to deny Me. Many well-meaning people, who have limits that are not everyone's limits, as well as personal denials that prevent the presence of full understanding have, even so, presented things that have value and intent to communicate. This is not what I am talking about here. They are sharing the extent of their knowledge while others are limiting the extent of knowledge they share. Being able to feel the difference here can show you that many things that appear to be the same are not necessarily the same. Everything that has claimed to have good intent, does not. Twists and turns on judgments are very prevalent in Earth's reality at this time. Judgment is already limiting, but judgment takes a more serious turn when it is twisted by the claim that it is fact, not judgment.

Medicine and science, for another example, have established the minimum daily requirements for certain nutrients without including in the spectrum that different people, vibrating at different rates and receiving different amounts of light in varying colors, need different nutrients in different amounts. Lifestyle, ancestral lineage, stress, pollution and every other variable are all factors to be taken into account here, too.

Every time a factor is rendered irrelevant, it is a form of judgment and denial. Reality is not something that should be delineated and defined in such limiting ways. These are attempts to lock up reality when reality is supposed to be fluid and evolving. Everything has consciousness and nothing is to be denied its role in Creation. The way in which most scientific experiments have been delineated renders them irrelevant to a free reality. The denials powering most of modern science have produced a reflection of their imbalances.

With few exceptions, schools have also been reinforcing and further programming the mass view of reality. Presenting a particular version of science and evolution as fact, while not accepting Creation as a participant in this is a twist and turn on judgments that is misleading to people. Even telling children that faerie-land exists only in stories, is giving them an image of reality that is based in many judgments. This denial does something worse than just disappointing children; it teaches them, from an early age, to deny what many of them see right in front of them. Most children have been convinced that many denials are true, when, in fact, they are not true. This is one of the many ways in which people have been taught to disconnect from the full spectrum of their own awareness and perceptions. This conditioning can make it difficult to suspend judgment and stop dismissing these things. One of the most direct ways to increase openness and widen the spectrum of awareness and perceptions is to start noticing, as much as you can, what you would usually ignore.

By starting with whatever you can notice first, which may be feelings you have generally dismissed as unacceptable, giving it as much acceptance and expression as you can, and by encouraging the listening, receiving and noticing aspects of your nature and expanding their expressive possibilities, you may be amazed at how your consciousness can expand and unfold into wider awareness. At present on Earth, everyday reality is both limiting possibilities and having its possibilities limited through patterns that have been held within rigid forms. These forms are not really reality. They are the images people have been projecting of reality, and there has been little awareness of the difference.

Churches and world religions that have been holding the image of themselves as having the best belief system have responsibility, here, as well. The images they promote are not the full picture. They are based in judgments that have been projected as fact. When churches and world religions hold beliefs in place about what I am, receptivity to My Loving Light can be limited by believing I must fit within the limited image of Me which they have accepted.

I am much more than what has been received on Earth so far. I am a living and evolving God. Belief systems reflect the ability to open and receive Me at the time they have been adopted. My Word has always been right for the time, place and situation of those receiving it. When people receive Me according to their own limitations, problems arise when those who may not have these same limitations do not question this or are intimidated into feeling that they dare not question this. Questioning has intent behind it, and should not all be labeled "doubt" or "lack of faith." As consciousness grows and expands, I can give more understanding. There is not a limit to this process. Images can become fluid, expand and align with one another. As consciousness

68

expands, more forms of truth, and deeper forms of truth, can be recognized.

The judgment that I am the same now as I was long ago and that I have nothing more to teach people than what was revealed long ago, are two of the judgments tied into the core of what has taken the spiral of evolution on Earth into the circular patterns of repetition. Externalizing judgments so that they are presented as fact instead of opinion, are major ways in which many judgments have been hidden.

When judgments become rigid forms, they can attempt to control everything and hold reality static within these limitations. This way of judging, without acknowledging that judgment is taking place, has become very prevalent and needs attention. Denials externalize parts of the self that will have to be recovered. Externalizing judgments and claiming they are not judgments, but reality, and further claiming that nothing can be done about it because it is just "the way it is," is a heavy denial of personal responsibility and of personal experience, reality and creative power. These denials carry deep-running currents that erode and wash away people's ability to create their own reality. Since these denials cannot be approached outwardly without receiving more denial, internal movement is necessary to reclaim these externalized parts of the self.

ACCEPTANCE

Form has been expressing imbalance because it expresses essence, and the essence of Spirit and Will have not been balancing in the Heart. Denial of the Spirit has caused many people to let judgments, and programming in their minds, run them. Denial of the Will has reinforced this, not only because the contributions of the Will cannot, then, participate in the mind's decisions, but also because the Spirit cannot be fully present if the Will is denied. Magnetic energy draws Spiritual energy into manifestation and holds it there. When the Will is denied, the Spirit is equally denied its full presence in manifestation.

The Will must open the space to receive the Spirit. To do this, the Will must feel from the Spirit unconditional, loving acceptance that allows it to freely vibrate. The essence of the Will wants to receive the Loving Light of Spirit. The Will must be allowed to express anything it needs to express in the process of manifesting unconditional acceptance of the Spirit. The Spirit and the Will must accept each other unconditionally. To do this yourself, you need to start where you are. Accept all of your feelings, and let them open your mind to accept more of your spiritual presence. If you have intent to find balance, do not let your mind continue to tell your Will how it should be feeling. The Will and the mind need to communicate in such a way that the imbalances can end. Agreement means that nothing is overpowering anything else. Being able to accept everything involved in the process of coming into agreement, without overpowering or denying anything, is the practice of *Right Use of Will*.

Many Spirits thought that they should experience and accept everything in Creation by becoming involved with it. These Spirits did not accept themselves first though. The self must unconditionally want to experience something before it is really the right experience for it. Instead, these Spirits overrode parts of themselves and pressured themselves to have these experiences. Any time acceptance is forced on a part of the self that does not have it, that part of the self either has to deny itself in favor of the experience or resist the experience. Often times, this resistant part of the self cannot stay totally present, and may even have to break off from the rest, if it cannot handle the overpowering. As this overriding of the self took place, these Spirits found themselves involved in things they could not handle. They were losing parts of themselves in these experiences, and other parts were leaving them. As this proceeded, confusion grew, and everything began to be more and more mixed up, so that it became more and more difficult to know if they were attracted to something, or not.

This practice of overriding parts of the self came from lack of experience, confusion between self and other and the nature of acceptance. The self must not diminish itself in favor of external experiences. A look at this path can show you that it leads to extinction. Having acceptance for the whole self will allow you to evolve into readiness for experiences or a willingness to see that they are not for you, at this time. In the very beginning, the Will pressured itself to accept light that did not feel loving to it by fearing that it was, itself, the problem by not being able to be loving or accepting enough to make a place for everything. If judgment is released about the initial response of the Will, space can be opened for change.

Will and Body are the parts of Spirit that enable Spirit to manifest on Earth. Believing that the Spirit had nothing to learn because it already knows everything, most Spirits judged against their Will and Body instead of accepting Them as their own manifested parts and realizing that They have their own way to learn in manifested experience. The Spirit cannot successfully pressure the Will to get ahead of itself because the Spirit thinks it should already be there. These misunderstandings greatly increased the pain and confusion in the Will. Acceptance allows the alignment necessary to have success in this learning experience.

Ending the denial of the Will includes accepting the pain the Will has had to hold. The question of how much pain your Will is likely to have to surface and process with your Spirit, depends on how much it has been having to hold because it was not allowed earlier release. Resistance to this indicates a need to release feelings of dislike, blame and even hatred toward the Will, often received by the Will as feelings of self-hatred. An understanding needed here, is that when there is a gap between feeling something and accepting those feelings, the energy generated in that gap is denial in some form. This has greatly diminished the manifestation of loving Spiritual presence on Earth

The Will has to have acceptance from the Spirit for whatever it needs to surface and express. In this way, it can release its held charge and become able to reach spontaneity, if the Spirit really helps. You can ask for My Presence to be there with you every time you feel yourself releasing old charge, and especially if something seems to be too much for you. Spiritual Healing and Amazing Grace are two of the ways people have explained how something that seemed insurmountable can suddenly be healed.

Events in your life, or what some call Karma, bring your patterns forward into experience so that you can see them. Mental recognition is not enough, though. When you hold parts of yourself apart and do not give them free expression and participation in the rest of your being, those places do not receive the benefits of this recognition. The understandings must reach all levels of your being. Experience is meant to teach so that people can evolve, but most people have been repeating patterns because they have not gained the needed understandings. The repetition that Karma allegedly brings has been because the understanding of everything involved has not yet been reached. The experiences come to try to bring another opportunity for you to find the understandings needed for you to evolve. Everything, including happiness, can evolve to greater heights. However, intent to evolve must be present and allowed to manifest.

Most people who have been saying that they have acceptance for their Karma, say this while not really looking at it. They are going through the motions of accepting whatever happens to them as though resigned to it, but haven't been learning much from their experiences. Karma is not a payment of debts to others so much as it is a manifestation of the person's held belief systems, judgments and limitations. Acceptance needs to be felt more fully, without the assumption that because it's being allowed, this means there is acceptance and surrender. If your true feelings do not want to accept or surrender, do not let it happen.

The image most people have been holding of surrender to God, My Will, or anything else it might be called, is not an accurate understanding. The image that joy can be found this way, if you just surrender more, is not accurate either. Holding an image of what you think is the correct spiritual attitude, rather than seeing what is really happening, holds true understanding away. The real truth for you is going to come from true self-acceptance and nowhere else. As you increase acceptance of your full self, you can gain more conscious ability to determine your reality. As it stands now, most people are being run by old Karma, or subconscious beliefs.

Trying to make themselves accept something when their Wills didn't like it, is just what happened when some Spirits became trapped on Earth in forms they didn't like. Most blamed their Wills. The feeling of being trapped, blamed and judged really opened the door to panic. This panic was overwhelming, and since it was not a pleasant feeling, the Spirits did not want to feel it. Instead of feeling and expressing them at the time, the Spirits largely suppressed their emotions here without realizing that not allowing free movement of their emotions was most of what was trapping them. These feelings need to be accepted now.

Earth people have been trying to accept reality as it is, but if they were to really feel their feelings, they would have to say that they don't like it much. The pain of the Will around this needs acceptance and not more judgment, dismissal, rejection or denial. Panic, deep fear and even terror are held undercurrent in most people and can be felt, if the depth of the true feelings is felt. In most people, these feelings have been hidden in shame, guilt and judgment because, at the core of it, has been the fear that being entrapped in this way had displeased My Loving Light. If you are starting to feel any of these feelings now, stop reading and let your feelings be felt; express and release everything that you can. Open to any further waves of these feelings also. These old feelings are the feelings of being trapped with no way out.

When you have released the judgments and given expression to the feelings that you are trapped with no way out, you will have made an opening to find one. Holding buried feelings of being powerless to help yourself impedes your ability to help yourself. Besides the intrinsic needs of the self, there is good reason to give these feelings acceptance, expression and release. The situation on Earth has been worsening and worsening because so many have been holding feelings that they can't do anything about it, and even that what is happening is deserved as punishment. This is really confusing the lesson with punishment.

As long as you believe you must accept something whether you like it or not, you are overriding your Will. If you are doing this to yourself, you are opening the door for others to do it to you, and perhaps more obscured from your view, also doing this to others. Overriding has been happening for a long time and has been heavily powered by many misunderstandings and denials. These misunderstandings and denials have been imprisoning the very emotional response that could change things for the better.

The situation on Earth is very perilous and needs immediate attention. It is actually to this point: The ones holding panic and terror, denied and not being given release, are as though against a wall or worse. The ones who have been denying these feelings are the ones who can help the situation by finding these suppressed and lost feelings within themselves, giving them expression and bringing them within the Light of Love. Hating these feelings and continuing to push them away, instead of allowing their movement as direct emotional expression, is going to precipitate more and more disastrous scenarios until events make it so that these feelings can no longer be held away from you, because they must break out of their entrapment somehow. Panic, fear, terror, anger and rage have the power to change these pictures if they are given loving acceptance and allowed direct expression as sounds and judgment release. Remember to ask for My Loving Light to come into these places that have been held outside of love. You may have taken on a guilt that says, since this is your own fault, you must accept punishment and fix it all by yourself. These feelings also need movement.

The feelings can become divinely attuned. The Will is attuned to the Destiny Path and is willing to undergo whatever is necessary to speed its recovery and seek fulfillment of its Destiny Path, but it needs loving acceptance to do this. If you are a Spirit of Loving Essence, you are a Spirit who can help the situation on Earth in this way. If you connect to these feelings and feel overwhelmed and out of control, even if you feel and express panic, fear, terror, anger and rage all at once, it is still better than any other option you have.

THE LAND OF PAN

I, now, want to tell some stories to help you understand more fully what I am talking about. These can be very enlightening stories and, if you can let yourself be triggered, helpful stories, also.

The popular version of the history of Earth is not entirely accurate and is another example of twists and turns on judgments. As I have said, many people have tried to avoid their responsibility on Earth in many ways. Pretending not to remember things that they have not wanted to remember is one of the main attempts at this, even to the extent of doctoring history so that it sounds better to the ones seeking to avoid responsibility. This has not really worked though, as quite a few people have felt that straightforwardness is lacking, and it is.

Many people have been denying so much that they have only a small, narrow opening through which information can be received. This has to be reversed now, because it has reached dangerous proportions on Earth. These stories of the past will help open your channels so that you can begin remembering what you have denied for so long.

In the beginning, when Spirits first entered the Earth, it was in a land called Pan, which is now under the Pacific Ocean. In the land of Pan, or Pangea, no one had to earn a living; everything sprang forth without effort. Every need was met by simply desiring it to be met, and the forms in which it was met often surprised and delighted the Spirits there. For example, a Spirit only needed to say, "I want to taste something good," and something delicious would appear, often in a form that had not been seen before. If a Spirit wished to experience immersing in water, a pool at just the desired temperature would appear, having all the things about it that this Sprit particularly liked. If a group of Spirits wished to swim, the pool would have everything everyone wanted.

In the beginning, many of the Spirits could change forms. Athough some had more mastery of this than others, all could do it. It was not unusual, at that time, for a Spirit to do acrobatics on the way to a pool with arms and legs, and then, upon diving into the water, transform legs into a fishtail if swimming was more fun in that form. If, later, there was a desire to fly, wings would appear. Some Spirits began taking this for granted. They received without feeling gratitude and even began to use these gifts to their own advantage. Hoarding of the abundance and the use of form to present the self as other than what it was, were two of the ways in which these gifts began to be abused.

Earth was created to be a living faerie-tale without any shadow of evil or doubt. The ones abusing the gifts did not know how to live on Earth, and many did not accept, or even like, Earth's intended way. They tried to make Earth Spirits feel that their faerie-land was silly, immature and just a pretend world. And to the Spirits denying Earth, it was a pretend world because they held a different view of reality within themselves. These Spirits had home planets other than Earth and were lost. They would not admit this, however. Instead, these Spirits acted superior and said they had come to protect Earth and all the Spirits who insisted on living in this silly faerie-tale with no protection from what was really going on in Creation.

Not long before this time, there had been a War in the Heavens. The faeries and elves, brownies and pixies, dwarves and gnomes, mermaids and all the other faerie folk on Earth had felt that the war was over. They were in a healing, celebrating mood. These other Spirits, who claimed they had come to protect them, did not want the war to be over. These Spirits had emerged during the War in the Heavens because they responded to that energy and started the fight.

The Earth Spirits had emerged earlier than these larger, fighting Spirits in a great burst of golden light, and had fallen away from Me before learning everything they had needed to know to be on their own. Some older Rainbow Spirits and some Angels, too, had gone after them to see if they could help because it didn't seem that they should already be on their own. All of these Spirits had come to Earth, and they all had one thing in common. They all had hidden feelings of rebelliousness toward Me. Many of them believed I had let lack of acceptance among my different kinds of Spirits go to unnecessary extremes, and that because I did not stop it, this had resulted in the War in the Heavens.

I want to give a short synopsis of what happened on Earth so that you can understand how the Earth came to be so dense and slow that magic seems lost, and manifesting and changing form seems difficult and slow. This is also how it happened that nearly everyone now feels they have to work for a living or inherit money. If Earth Spirits feel their true feelings, they feel that Earth is not the way it was meant to be, but that everything has become a trade-off or a compromise, instead.

Long ago, in Pan, the air smelled of flowers, and the Earth was soft with mosses, grasses and sandy beaches. The rocks were gemstones, and the waters were liquid light that sparkled and danced. The weather, and even the seasons, changed in reflection of the moods of the Spirits. This harmony manifested as music. Even the wind in the trees and the waves on the seas gave rhythm to the melodies. The monkeys and cats and all the birds sang and danced with the faerie folk. The fish and the mermaids even sang in the seas. Everything glowed with colored light during the golden day and also during the soft, blue night. Desire manifested reality so easily that a Loving Spirit could extend a hand toward a tree and that tree would flower immediately. Reality appeared to change magically, affected by every Spirit's feelings of how it should be.

I have to speak lyrically here because Pan was so magical, musical and free and is what many faerie-tales are based on. The Spirits there allowed entry of many Spirits who claimed they wanted to be a part of this reality, but many of these Spirits only came to disagree with them about how Earth should be. They invaded Earth and claimed they did not. These were fighting Spirits who said they were Warriors sent by Me. The rebellious ones had too much fear to ask Me to make it clear. They feared that I was angry with them for leaving Me too soon. They feared the Spirits who were telling them they were wrong were speaking for Me. They dreaded and feared that they deserved punishment.

These faerie folk did not know these Warriors had another place they were supposed to go. They did not understand that these Warriors would create conflict wherever they went because conflict was what had called them forth. These Warriors claimed they were just in the nick of time to hold the line against danger that was lurking all around and protect these childish Spirits who were refusing to see what actually lurked hidden in everything they could see.

In fact, these Warriors did find danger and strife lurking wherever they looked because that was how they wanted it to be, and that was all that they could see. The more the Warriors claimed to be finding danger on Earth, the more the other Spirits began to fear that the Warriors really had reason to be there. The more the Earth Spirits began to fear, the harder it became for them to stay clear. They no longer felt sure that joy and freedom had much allure, if they were being naïve about danger lurking near. Some even feared that struggle and strife were a necessary part of Me and of life.

These Spirits also had fear that they had to listen to these Warriors because they couldn't depend on Me anymore or on what they thought Creation was meant to be. They even thought I didn't look much to Earth because they weren't interesting to Me, and that what they were doing didn't have much worth. Judgments were made here that changed their reality. It was no longer considered appropriate to be creative, wild and free; everyone now was supposed to be orderly. The Warriors reflected these fears by saying the Earth Spirits wouldn't be hearing directly from Me anymore. They said I had sent them as My emissaries and intermediaries, to head up Earth, implement My orders and protect them from realities full of hidden dread. They were lying, but the Earth Spirits didn't suspect this at first.

In this way, step by step, the Warriors began to lead the Spirits on Earth exactly where they dreaded to be. Everyone on Earth still tried to be gay and free, and play and say they still could live in their old way. The Warriors said that they had saved the day; the Earth Spirits felt they couldn't be sure. The Warriors wanted Earthlings to live by rules, "Because," they said, "we can't protect unpredictable fools."

The head of the Warriors then began to say there were so many marauding Spirits flying around that we need more protection than what has already been found. He was not completely wrong either, for as long as the Warriors were there, there was always going to be something to fear. They have a purpose in My Creation, and I am not unloving toward them, but Earth is no longer their right place.

The head Warrior called for more protection, over and over, more and more, so loud and long that Earth finally answered the call by placing some protective fire dragons in the skies. These fire dragons had taken on an intimidating form that was huge enough to encircle the Earth. They hung out in the skies, watching everything with very sharp eyes. With their breath of fire, they blew away Spirits they didn't want to enter the Earth, but they didn't remove any that were already there. They did not believe that they could or should, and so, denied their true feelings there. There were many on Earth that they wanted to send away, but feared it was wrong and that they might scorch others who got in the way. If they had accepted their own true feelings, they could have found a way. Instead, the fire dragons held in many of their true feelings and only expressed towards Spirits trying to enter for the first time.

These denied feelings became dense within them because they were not allowed to move. When their density caused them to sink toward Earth, they began to take turns in the sky while the others went to the fire seas, deep in the Earth, to purify themselves of what had made them too dense to hang in the skies. They got there through secret and guarded passageways that opened only to the fire dragons. In the fire seas, the fire dragons vented their feelings, which often meant dumping them out.

While the fire dragons regularly purified, their denied and pushed away feelings opened the way for one among them to become treacherous and foul. In actuality, this fire dragon feared his own worth and had externalized this as right place issues of power and position. He interpreted right place in My Creation as a judgment of worth, which it is not. This fire dragon saw self-worth as who had the most important place.

He actually wanted to take My place, but he planned to begin by awarding himself what he saw as the most important power position on Earth. He decided he was going to make himself "head fire dragon." He wanted to be the one to say who could come and go from Earth, but he disguised his true purpose by saying that "No one should judge this way. Instead, let all Spirits enter; let all Spirits stay,"

He did not feel good to the other fire dragons, and his words did not ring true, but the fire dragons' own denials did not let them know what to do. He implied that he was more loving than they. He said they were judging him and the others who wanted to be on Earth. His presence was intimidating to the other fire dragons who did not know what to do. He had become the biggest, and he turned his fire on them, which none of the others did. Fearing they dared not speak up, the others vented underground, when this fire dragon was not around. They wanted to tell him to leave Earth. Instead, they asked him to leave, and he refused. He was asked not to allow any Spirit onto Earth unless the other fire dragons approved. The fire dragons wanted consensus, and again, he refused.

Meanwhile, the Warriors began refusing to protect Earth for free. They began to demand gifts and services. Without admitting that they could not manifest like the others, the Warriors insisted that tribute was their just do. In this way, they were using the light of others, instead of receiving from Me. Whatever they received from the Earth Spirits, they saw as not being what they wanted it to be. When they received something, gratitude was missing. They all complained that it was not enough, and the more they complained, the more they decided they needed to demand for themselves. Their power issues wanted complete control. The Warriors demanded everything as their just do, and still, they felt empty and incomplete and as though what they were receiving wasn't enough.

The Earth Spirits felt they were having to agree to more and more control and less and less abundance for themselves. They had fear, which many covered with anger. Their fears about Me did not allow them to ask for My help. They called out My Name and said they were asking for My help, but greatly feared they would hear nothing, or that I would not give them the answers they wanted to hear. They beseeched Me for help, and I did not answer. The Earth Spirits feared, even more then, that I had sent the Warriors in My place.

I did not send the Warriors, but I also could not lift this struggle off of Earth. The Warriors had their own viewpoint in place of hearing Me. Other Spirits who had gone to Earth to try and help, found that they, also, felt unreceived and far away from My Light. There was growing confusion and fear, and the treacherous fire dragon planned to take advantage of the situation. He suggested that they would all feel better if they had a big party and invited all to forget their differences and celebrate what they had. He even volunteered to guard Earth alone that night so that the other fire dragons could go to the party.

The other fire dragons did not trust him. They decided they'd take turns guarding with him that night. One of the fire dragons, though, could not stand being on duty with this treacherous one. When it was his turn, he left his post and slunk off to the fire seas, telling himself everyone was so busy partying that no one would notice. He did not feel good about doing this, but his own denials did not allow him to find another way to exercise what he thought was his own free Will.

The treacherous fire dragon had a plan and had been hoping there would be a time when he could be alone in the sky. This fire dragon had been communing with another force that opposed Me, and as soon this fire dragon was alone in the sky, he called to that force and let it onto Earth. He thought that he was about to gain control of all of Earth because he thought he could control this force and have it intimidate Earth for him.

This force, however, had another Spirit already controlling it that this fire dragon had not seen because of his power delusions. This Spirit blasted past the fire dragon with that force, and hit Earth with its hot, dry, raging, cosmic wind of destructive anger. The fire dragon, who had thought he was about to take over, was scorched and thrown to Earth like a discarded rag doll. He was barely able to crawl into a cave and hide himself. Writhing in agony, he tried to abandon his form to escape his pain.

This hot, dry wind raged across the face of Pan that night and sent the partying ones scurrying for shelter. It burned off vegetation, seared great cracks into the land, and made it unbearably hot and steamy on Earth. Its raging fingers reached into the Earth itself causing volcanoes and earthquakes. The hot dry wind could not stay in one place; it raged on, wreaking destruction everyplace it went, until, finally, it seemed to burn out.

At first, the Earth Spirits feared that it was Me who had hit Earth to punish. Then, some thought the fire dragons must have done this, but when they sought the fire dragons and asked them, the ones they found claimed they didn't know anything about it. When they found the treacherous one, he claimed he had suffered terribly trying to defend Earth. The other one, who was supposed to be on guard with him, said that he had been hurt, too. The Earth Spirits now had even more fear of Me because they did not know how the hot, dry wind had come to Earth. They did not know if it would return or not. They feared they could not depend on anything. The head Warrior said that the existing protection was obviously not enough.

The Earth recovered from this as best it could, but the land was not as abundant or as beautiful as it had been. As the Spirits healed themselves and the Earth, they tried to return to their own ways and find some joy again. Even so, they had scars they weren't able to heal yet. In seeking their old ways, they also sought old friends, and when many of them could not be found, they felt a growing sense of things not being right on Earth. The Spirits of Earth had not encountered death before, and they did not know what they were encountering then, but they had a persistent feeling that they needed to find their friends to know what had happened to them.

In their search, they found a Spirit on Earth who had not been there before. When the Earth Spirits of Pan found him, they did not know what he was or what he was doing, but they knew that they feared him. He said he was a powerful wizard who had come to Earth to help heal Earth because he had experience with the hot, dry wind. He lied here. He did not come to heal the Earth, but he did have experience with the hot, dry wind; he was its master. He told them that the hot, dry wind was all that was left of an entire universe that had destroyed itself with the raging fire of its own destructive anger.

The dark wizard sought to gain control of Earth. He had seen that it could serve his purpose to hit Earth with this hot, dry wind, and thus, bring this destructive anger to Earth and fan its flames into another inferno. He also had to increase the density of Earth quickly, or he could not stay. In trying to shrink away from the attack of the hot, dry wind, the Earth, and everything on it, had increased its density. As soon as he arrived on Earth, the dark wizard began to ceaselessly frighten every Spirit into shrinking away from him in denial of the reality he had brought to Earth. He set about squelching everything expansive, and he had helpers.

I want you to know that the dark wizard is about to find himself removed from the Earth because his flames of destructive anger have reached the potential for nuclear holocaust. He cannot succeed in destroying the Earth because the Earth itself does not want to be destroyed. I will tell you more, now, about what the dark wizard did to gain control in Pan.

The dark wizard unabashedly told everyone that their missing friends had been eaten. When he saw their horrified response, he denied their horror by saying everyone had accepted this on his planet because they knew how to share energy and become one with each other in a way that Earth hadn't learned yet. He acted more knowing than anyone and said that it was only fair to take turns being and being food for those who were being. He said it was time for Earth to do this.

The dark wizard had brought with him many Spirits who had not been on Earth before. These Spirits had entered forms already present on Earth. As the dark wizard spoke, he pointed his finger at some of these Spirits, and beings who had not done this before began fighting, killing and eating each other. This was frightening and strange. Until then, no one on Earth had ever eaten anything other than what had manifested solely to be eaten. No one had overpowered another against their Will to this extent on Earth before. These Spirits were fighting, overpowering others and disappearing them by eating them. The Spirits being eaten were screaming with pain and terror. This traumatized the Spirits on Earth.

The dark wizard said they were screaming in ecstasy and denied that any of these Spirits had overpowered the forms they had entered. He said that they were well-received because many wanted to learn this lesson. The Warriors liked fighting, and even though they maintained a stoic presentation, the Earth Spirits feared that the Warriors liked this. The Earth Spirits felt very alone and afraid. The dark wizard denied everything the Earth Spirits felt here by saying that these beings were only becoming one with each other. Then, he said, "How could it be overpowering? It's impossible to overpower anyone against their Will."

He was right, but only if there is no denial present. Once denial of true feelings got started, it increased until it began to overwhelm the very Spirits who had thought denial would protect them from being overwhelmed. In the beginning of Pan, denial was not extensive. The dark wizard had his work cut out for him. He did not mind though; he was driven by rage and hatred for Me and My Creation. He was intent on increasing denial and density as much as he could, and the Spirits he brought with him helped him do this. I call these Spirits "denial Spirits" because denial fuels them. These Spirits had been helping the denial wizard everywhere he went. Now, on Earth they began helping him deny everything that could be denied.

At first, they began by telling everyone things that undermined their free Will. I will give you an example of their approach, and you will have to do your homework on this. If a denial Spirit were to lie down on a path through the woods, and another Spirit came running, hopping, skipping and jumping along, the denial Spirit would jump up and scream, "You cannot come running right through the place where I am lying!"

If the other Spirit said, "I'm sorry. This is a path, and I wasn't expecting you to be lying there," without any acknowledgment that he might be the one who needs to move, the denial Spirit would say, "Sorry isn't enough! You might have stepped on me! Find another path!"

If the Spirit said it would not have stepped on the other Spirit because it would have noticed in time, the denial Spirit would

82

have denied the Earth Spirit's sensitivity, attunement, ability to notice in time and anything else it could deny on the spot. If the Spirit did anything other than abdicate to the denial Spirit, the denial Spirit would continue to deny everything presented to it.

When some Earth Spirits tried telling these denial Spirits to leave, they denied their right to do this, claiming they had been there all along and had as much right to be on Earth as anyone else. What they said was true, as far as it went. Denial had been there all along, unrecognized, but these Spirits only mentioned what furthered them, and there were many things about the situation that the Spirits on Earth were afraid to look at very closely, let alone feel. It was very upsetting to them to remember much of what had happened around the hot, dry wind or the Spirits who had begun to fight, kill and eat one another. They doubted their own perceptions and wondered how much had been happening all along that they hadn't let themselves notice.

I have seen and heard all of this, and I have understanding and acceptance of denial Spirits. Denial Spirits cannot do anything with you unless you have denial they can use. Since Earth had denial happening already, these Spirits had an opportunity to gain a foothold. In gaining a foothold, they had an opportunity to increase the denial on Earth, and because of the unseen role of denial, the Spirits on Earth were not able to resolve this.

I have studied denial Spirits for a long time in order to understand them, and I am having to teach this to Earth because Earth has become very confused by the presence of so many denial Spirits. Every kind of Spirit has had to face denial Spirits. Denial Spirits have taken every form there is and reflected the denial of every kind of Spirit. Denial gave form to these Spirits, and when denial ends, these Spirits will no longer be present on Earth. In the meantime, as you end your own denials, they will trouble you less and less.

If the Spirit on the path in the woods had had no denial, he would not have gotten entangled in any denial there. He could have continued running, leaped over the denial Spirit and been gone. In this case, the Earth Spirit's denials had grown big enough that the denial Spirit had become an intimidating form. There were many denials present there, but the imbalance My Light wants to mention now is that not wanting anyone to spoil his good time had become turned around in this Spirit to not thinking it was alright to spoil anyone else's good time.

Then, the Spirits on Earth did not have enough experience to know who was meant to be on Earth and who was not. Because there has been both denial Spirits and Loving Essence mistakenly denied, many Spirits on Earth have been confused about how they really feel here, and have tried to figure out how they should feel. Ending your own denials is going to allow you to sort this out.

Those who do not belong on Earth are being directed by My Light to their right place. Everything has its right place, where it's not any problem to be the way it is. Everyone on Earth has had misunderstandings about loving acceptance that caused them to think they had to pressure themselves to accept things they did not like and refrain from expressing any other feelings about it. Only now have Earth Spirits seen enough to be able to understand this. Then they tried to accept everything as just another Spirit's way. The basic denial that allowed denial Spirits to take advantage of Earth was denial of Me. My Presence was denied here. For a long time, I have not been able to give the understandings I wanted to give. I need to give them now.

After the original entry of the hot, dry wind and the denial wizard's introduction of physical death through overpowering, the Spirits in Pan experienced another event that greatly increased denial. The denial wizard began challenging everyone to "duels of magic," as he called them. There were many wizards on Earth, then, and, for the most part, only wizards accepted his challenges. The denial wizard defeated everyone who accepted his challenge. He won by denying the validity of the other wizards' approaches and insisting that the duels had to be conducted according to his rules.

A number of wizards saw his duel for what it was and refused his challenge. Some of these wizards saw him gaining power on Earth and thought that he must be stopped. There were also many other Spirits on Earth who feared he was gaining power and wanted him stopped. Others denied their fear by saying that he wasn't such a bad guy after all. Some said his power gain was only an illusion that they weren't going to believe in.

Spirits increased their denial in many ways and looked at less of what was really happening on Earth because they did not like seeing and feeling what the denial wizard was doing. This gave the denial wizard a lot of space and a lot of denial energy on which to feed. He became more and more powerful, and began to be more outrageous, too. He found he could do things right in front of others that they did not want to see, and they did not see them. If he was noticed, he denied what he was actually doing and said he was doing something else. Some, who didn't want to accept the horror of what was happening, actually helped the dark wizard by explaining away his outrages.

Finally, one wizard stepped forward and answered the challenge of the dark wizard because he strongly felt the need to get this denial wizard off of Earth. This wizard had studied the other duels of magic, and he had a plan. Because he had noticed how the dark wizard denied everything offered to him, this wizard thought the dark wizard would refuse any terms offered to him. He offered the dark wizard everything that he did not really want him to agree to. This wizard did not realize, however, just how extensive the dark wizard's denial really was. The dark wizard immediately recognized the light wizard's denial. Instead of denying the denial offer, the dark wizard accepted this light wizard's denial of himself and insisted he stick to the deal.

The dark wizard was not like the light wizard. The light wizard had looked at the dark wizard closely, but he had not seen him thoroughly. He had misjudged his denial, and he had misjudged his scruples; he thought he actually had some and gave the dark wizard the benefit of the doubt. The light wizard had seen another thing inaccurately there, also. He had seen himself defeating the dark wizard and his own power ascending on Earth, but said he was doing this for the benefit of everyone else. He had that part of himself invested in this future, and so that part was not in the present. He had seen other possibilities, too, and had ignored all of them in favor of his favorite choice. Not realizing he needed to withdraw his emotional energy from these unpleasant possibilities, he had cut them off, leaving a part of himself there, also.

The light wizard had fear of this duel of magic because he felt he'd been trapped already into doing something he now felt he did not want to do. He could not admit this because he had too much pride. This wizard also had some stage fright about doing his feats of magic in front of everyone on Earth at once. The stakes were so high it was no longer just for fun. He had accepted though, so he felt he had to do it. In not allowing his fears, he had denied them.

On the day of the duel, the light wizard arrived on the scene early and paced up and down, waiting for the dark wizard. Many Spirits were already crowding into the area when the dark wizard arrived. The dark wizard only acknowledged denial, so he did not acknowledge many of the Spirits who were there. Although he didn't understand the impact of his own denial, and did not call it denial, the light wizard feared denial and, for the most part, really wanted to help Earth.

The light wizard began the duel of magic by hurling lightening bolts into the air. The dark wizard responded by drying up a lake and withering trees. The light wizard did not like this, but according to the rules, he was not allowed to complain. The light wizard feared the dark wizard was using these duels as an opportunity to do additional harm to a lot of things on Earth.

The light wizard was trying to think of what he could do that would not give the dark wizard an opportunity to do harm, when the dark wizard began accusing him of being too slow. He announced that if the light wizard was so slow, he probably couldn't do it. All the denial Spirits chimed in on this. The other Spirits thought it was unkind and unfair to ridicule anyone, so they did not say anything at all except some encouragement for the light wizard that was drowned out in the ruckus.

The dark wizard pressured the light wizard to hurry up. The light wizard suggested that they go immediately into form changes, thereby turning things inward instead of onto the Earth. The light wizard changed himself into a succession of animals and ran around doing everything they would do. He returned to his own form and received the applause of many Spirits who loved him.

The dark wizard smiled a superior smile, and said he would not stoop to such silliness. He insisted that the light wizard try something really difficult. Otherwise, it wasn't even a duel of magic, as far as he was concerned. The light wizard felt very denied here and said that if his form changes were so easy, the dark wizard should do it. The dark wizard scoffed, and as he stood there scoffing, he slowly turned himself into a black stone. The light wizard was aghast because he dreaded that particular challenge.

The light wizard knew that the validity of anything he did, other than turning himself into a stone, was going to be denied by the dark wizard and made to look silly. He did not want to argue with the dark wizard and let it be known that he was afraid. He pondered what to do and decided he would have to try it. He felt quite sure he could turn himself into a stone, but he didn't know if he could get back out of it. He told himself that he must do this or look like the loser.

While the light wizard was thinking all of this, the dark wizard returned to his wizard form. The light wizard knew the time had come for his turn. He pressured himself to change into the form of a stone, against his Will. He denied his fear, and pressured and pressured himself until he finally turned into a bluish, amethyst-like crystal.

The light wizard, then, got stuck in the stone because he did not know how to get himself moving again. His fear of the compression had made matters worse. He had believed that he could not express his fears and also win the duel of magic at the same time, so he had denied his fear, which was considerable, and this had put him over the midpoint. In one afternoon, the light wizard went from seeing himself as the most powerful wizard on Earth into finding himself trapped in a stone.

The light wizard was fearing, suffocating and panicking in the stone, and still, he could not get out. In his panic, he sensed My presence there, trying to help him get out of the stone. He refused My help because he was too frightened, too panicked and too confused to be sure it was Me or realize that there was any possibility at that time other than having to face everyone and be declared the loser of the duel of magic. He feared that he had let Me down. He thought I was also judging him, and there in the stone, the light wizard was judging himself very heavily.

The dark wizard ridiculed and belittled the light wizard and pronounced himself the winner of the duel. The dark wizard's supporters jeered at the light wizard just as he had believed they would.

I did not see the duel of magic as a struggle between good and evil, but on Earth it was seen as this. Even in the stone, the light wizard could feel the fear the Earth Spirits had that the dark wizard could get control of Earth. He felt that anything he could do now was after the fact. He felt that he had let all of Earth down. Stuck in the stone there, the light wizard was so overwhelmed by his emotions that he tried to split himself off from his pain in any way that he could. He wrenched as much of himself out of the stone as he could and left the rest there. His worst pain remained in the stone. This part needs to be recovered for the light wizard to recover his full presence on Earth.

The light wizard left so much of himself in the stone that, even though this part of him managed to emerge, no one recognized him except the dark wizard, who saw what others were afraid to see. The dark wizard immediately pounced on this fragment of the light wizard, overpowered him while he was still disoriented and devoured him in full view of everyone, yet, no one seemed to see it. As the dark wizard began to walk away, his helpers picked up the stone that was still there and followed behind him.

Only those who ran and hid were able to escape the aftermath of this duel of magic. While they managed to escape further direct experience with the dark wizard, they could not escape all of their feelings and, so, took with them whatever effect the duel had had on them. Whether they had denial of their fear or not, all the Spirits who saw what happened to the light wizard in the duel of magic now had fear struck into their Hearts.

The light wizard lost the duel to his own denials before he even began the duel of magic, but the misunderstanding at that time was that he had been overpowered by the dark wizard, himself. This misunderstanding gave the dark wizard a lot of power he would not otherwise have had. He had successfully created the illusion of having overpowered the light wizard with his own power. He has continued to do this ever since.

The dark wizard has also continued to be a master of form change and has remained powerful because of people's denial. He needs to leave Earth soon, but he cannot leave until his stolen power has been taken back from him by the ones who gave it to him with their denials and their belief that he had more power than they did. There are many judgments about power that need release here, too. He is going to go to his right place, but I do not want him to take any denied essence of loving Spirits with him.

I want all of you to end your denial so that neither you, nor any part of you, goes where he is going. If there are some places in you that do not feel like they belong to you, let Me have the final word here by accepting My need to put everything in its right place. Accepting and letting go can be protected if you ask Me to help you by putting everything in its right place. Then the dark wizard can go to his right place with only his own energy, and you will have all that is yours with you. I have to tell you that if you are not ready to let go of denial and accept yourself, you will have to go wherever your denial takes you. The fear involved here may see this as threatening you, but this is not My intent. I am the One who has been, and still is, warning you. I am telling you what is happening, but I am not telling you it has to happen to you. You have free Will. I am explaining what denial creates.

The rest of what I want to say about Pan, right now, is going to give more understandings about the denial present on Earth today. The Spirits having fear of the dark wizard held this fear within themselves and did not express it because they did not have the self-acceptance or understandings they needed. They tried to live their life the way they had been living it before the duel of magic took place. In order to do this, they had to deny many feelings, especially fear. Then, they repeated the pattern of the light wizard. They all tried to continue doing what they had been doing, and in trying to change form, they all got themselves stuck to varying degrees in varying forms. When they tried to get out, they found that they had to do it in the same way that the light wizard had had to do it. They did not understand how it could be that the dark wizard had so much power over them. They did not realize that they were doing this to themselves.

The dark wizard, of course, had no problem taking the credit. He was at work trying to increase his power in any way he could, and if other Spirits wanted to help him do it, he saw that his methods were working. He increased himself this way until he was looking more powerful than anyone else on Earth. He was so obnoxious to the Spirits who did not like his ways that the only ones who wanted to go near him were those who shared his insatiable lust for control and power over others. This reflection gave Earth Spirits many more judgments that need to be looked at now.

I did not intervene, then, because I saw that these experiences were necessary in order to gain certain understandings, and yet, I have felt the pain of everyone involved. I know all of you on Earth very well, and I could see that even though you had pain and suffering, you had to learn for yourselves why sacrifice, or denial of yourself in favor of others, does not work.

Pan changed after this duel of magic. It was still very beautiful by any of today's standards, but it now had a more dense form of light. The manifestations and changes took longer, and they all took more effort. Instead of calling a reality to them, Spirits now found it easier to go to that reality. Certain settings began to settle into certain places on Earth, and Spirits who were having trouble agreeing on their surroundings, solved it by leaving the surroundings in one place and going back there when they wanted to.

Many Spirits who still wanted the freedom of form changes began having trouble doing it. Many got stuck in forms that limited them in ways they had never before been limited. In many cases, Spirits who thought they desired a particular form in the moment in which they had entered it, now had difficulty in changing the form when the Spirit no longer wanted to remain in that form. Denial was the reason here, also. Denial of the fear that the dark wizard had power on Earth was only part of it. The denial that allowed him on Earth to begin with, was another part of it. The dark wizard had no more power than he was handed, but he was taking full advantage of everything that came his way.

The fragmenting of Spirits that was taking place when they had to get out of something the way the light wizard did, was taking many Spirits in Pan close to their midpoint. The fear around this loss of power was not given the acceptance it needed. Instead, these fears were denied, and blame began to be placed. Some Spirits blamed My lack of presence, some blamed others and many blamed the dark wizard. Almost everyone involved blamed themselves to a certain extent, and in doing that, put the blame on the part of themselves that they felt had caused the problem. Some blamed their Spirit and Me. Others blamed their feelings, or Will. Many who blamed the Will said that instead of accepting everything, it had resisted, and resistance had caused the problem. Many on Earth didn't dare to blame Me, but blamed their own Spirits, instead, in these same ways.

One part of the self blaming another part of the self caused a split in the consciousness. The warring in some individuals between their own Spirit and Will has been very extensive. Many people have even disconnected as totally as they can from parts of themselves. This diminished the Spiritual presence on Earth of everyone involved, even more. The denial reached such extensive proportions that physical death began to result. When Spirits felt that they could not get any farther with their own Wills and the forms in which they were enmeshed, they began volitionally breaking off from parts of themselves for a while and returning later to work on realigning themselves. This began the pattern of death and reincarnation, or of focusing consciousness into different levels of existence at different times.

The reality is that Body and Will do not completely lose awareness during the time their Spirit is not with Them, but They do lose the ability to express or understand it. You need to know that anything that has ever happened to any part of you will have to be accepted into your consciousness. Because it has happened to you, it cannot be denied. It is important to realize this in its full implication. Denial of what has been happening to Body and Will on Earth has been very strong and really needs attention.

Denial must be recognized in order for it to end. The longer you wait to end your denial, the more denial there will be for you to clear. Many have tried to deny that they have any denial in order to avoid the overwhelming reality they would feel if they accepted it. Many have tried to avoid the impact of what they have really done by telling themselves that God wouldn't really let this happen. I had to let this happen, and I will tell you why now. You would not listen to Me. Nothing less than the experience of everything that has happened to you on Earth was going to get the understandings across to you or you would have them already. And, in fact, many will not hear Me yet.

I am having to intervene now as I eventually had to, long ago in Pangea. I intervened, then, because I had to straighten things out enough that Spirits could go on and try to resolve this for themselves. When I projected a part of Myself onto Earth in the land of Pan to intervene personally, I found every sort of possible confusion of form that Earth could have come up with then. All that needed human form and would accept help from Me at that time, received a human form in which to work out their situation on Earth. I also made some rules to protect form from chaos until form could be better understood on Earth. A rule I made then was that animals and humans could not join their forms together, and could not mate and have children together. Prior to this rule, everything had been mixing together and forms had been going rapidly toward chaos.

Though I intervened, I did not remove the dark wizard from Pangea, and though he has had only the power to use denial, I will emphasize again that he took advantage of everything that came his way. Denial has been increasing on Earth ever since these times. I am intervening again because denial has again been crossing the midpoint. I am going to bring another form to Earth that will help you work out your situation. This form is called for because there is now enough experience that it can be accepted; this form is the form of right place.

I now want to go on and follow these experiences through two subsequent civilizations on Earth that also had My intervention. I stepped in to restore the balance point because it was necessary, and that is what I am having to do now.

LEMURIA

The split and disconnection that took place between the Spirit and the Will during the time of Pan led to the next two major experiences on Earth. Lemuria polarized to the Will, Atlantis polarized toward the Spirit, and both civilizations tried to prove that their polarity was superior.

The Will felt very hurt over being blamed for the problems in Pan. Feeling it could not rely on Spirit, the Will felt it was going to have to go on, on its own. Ultimately, this is not really possible, but the attempt was a necessary experience. Because of the judgments present, the Will in Lemuria was not able to receive the Loving Light of Spirit, release their pain over what had happened and reconnect with their Spirit there.

Lemurians called their land the Motherland. Many of the Spirits whose home planet is the Earth, lived in Lemuria. The name Lemuria calls lemurs to mind, but the Lemurians were not lemurs. The people were small and brown, slender and lithe, but they had no tail, and they were not covered with hair. Although the Will still held a great deal of pain there, the split between Spirit and Will had given the Lemurians a feeling of freedom from what they had been experiencing as the admonishing presence of Spirit, and not feeling continually judged, they were able to evolve the Will to a high degree. They enjoyed this time of feeling as though they had more self-acceptance, but they also had feelings they held in the background that feared this was not alright with My Light and that they were going to be punished for this.

Lemuria had a lovely civilization in its height. It was set in a subtropical garden that had no insects or reptiles. Flowers and fruits were everywhere for the picking, and no one ever had to think about how daily needs were gong to be met. Everyone made sure that everyone was well taken care of and had a place in the housing compounds. These compounds were much like Spanish haciendas that enclosed lovely gardens in the middle. They were plastered white with a plaster that resisted the subtropical rains. Pottery was a developed art and so was fresco painting. Groups of people often made combinations of the plentiful foods available, served them in large pottery dishes and offered them to everyone around. They made baskets and soft mattings for sleeping. The Lemurians had whatever clothing they wanted for fun and adornment, but clothing wasn't a necessity for them. The Lemurians were again able to feel like children playing and having fun, and they often made music and danced for hours every day.

They were happy to be recovering again and felt they could do anything they willed themselves to do. They could teleport themselves with the power of their Will, but they also enjoyed leaping, jumping and soaring. They were natural acrobats and were more adept than any monkey in the trees and vines. There were also others in Lemuria to whom I had given human form, however, many were people who had been trapped in the monkey family in Pan. There they had learned just what monkeys do, and later had been restored to a fuller consciousness, in part as a result of their acceptance of the state of consciousness they had inhabited in monkey forms.

The Lemurians learned to do many things with sound directed by the Will, including moving of rocks and other things, some sculpture and healing if anyone had the need. They had spiritual beliefs of a Mother in the Heavens, who, together with their Father had made this home for them. They acknowledged that they had a Father, and many of the things they did were because of the presence of My Loving Light that did love the Will, but they related more directly to the Divine Presence of a Mother and longed for Her warm embrace. Spiritual teachings were given to everyone, and many understandings, since lost about the Will, were known then, and taught. Their Hearts were open, especially to the Will energy, so they were very warm, as was their climate, but not wanting any more loss, they were also possessive. They had close ties with others, pride in their Will orientation, their way of life and in the ways they were developing.

The Lemurians were able to recover much of their lost understanding, but not all of it. They were a very high people though, and they were very joyful and loving and accepting of everything, except their own Spirits, which they felt had judged them and abandoned them to their earlier entrapment. They felt they had evolved out of their predicament in Pan without the help of their Spirits, and not having felt helped by their Spirits, they did not feel very inclined to let their Spirits come back and reap the benefits of their recovery.

They did acknowledge that My Light had helped them, though, and because of the presence of My Light, the Lemurian culture spiraled higher and higher in its evolvement. However, without their own Spirit's presence to help them grow and evolve, the Lemurians began to exhaust their possibilities. If they had been able to find acceptance then, Lemurians could have healed this polarization between their Wills and their Spirits, but it did not happen. Neither side was ready to release their viewpoint. Instead, the judgments were made over and over again.

Lemurians refused anything that felt judgmental toward their polarity. Will was being reactive and, yet, at the same time, was feeling its own potential and beauty. Lemurians had a long time to see what they could do, but they still didn't open very much to their own Spirit presence. Most Lemurians continued to be distrustful of Spirit, and, from their viewpoint, not without reason.

In the height of Lemuria, some teachers came to teach Lemurians about the Spirit. Even though these teachers claimed to have come from Me to help Lemuria, most Lemurians were suspicious of the teachers' motives and distrusted their teachings. While most of the teachers saw themselves as only trying to help Lemurians accept the Spirit, the Lemurians felt that the teachers were trying to frighten and control them. The teachers were met with lack of receptivity, and even defensiveness. The Lemurians felt that these teachers had undercurrent judgments against them and against their ways. They felt they were being subtly criticized and told they were wrong.

Some of these teachers did have judgments that the Lemurians were not receptive, did not want help and refused to learn. Some judged that the Lemurians were upsetting them and were not right to do this. When their teachings were refused, some, however, judged that they weren't good teachers. Some judged that they were upsetting the people and should leave them to their own ways. Undercurrent here, though, was an anger that said they would soon learn the folly of their own ways. There were many judgments made by these teachers against the Lemurians and against themselves, and the Lemurians also made judgments about the teachers and, also, themselves. Most of these judgments were reiterations of earlier judgments made by their own Spirits telling their Wills they should be doing better, or differently, than they were and the Wills reacting to blame themselves and/or their Spirits.

Together, then, the Lemurians and those who came to help them, created an atmosphere that, for the most part, increased the polarization, rather than helping it. No amount of effort was able to succeed in bridging the gap there. Then, dinosaurs began to appear in Lemuria. Having already devastated everything in their path, the dinosaurs had eaten their way to the Lemurian settlements. When dinosaurs first began to appear in Lemuria, most Lemurians felt the teachers had drawn them. The teachers, for the most part, didn't see themselves as responsible for the dinosaurs. They saw the Lemurians as having drawn this.

When the dinosaurs came to Lemuria, many Lemurians were afraid that I had sent them as punishment. Many thought the teachers shared the blame for desiring punishment for the Lemurians. Some of the Lemurians tied some of these teachers to trees as sacrifices to the dinosaurs. When these teachers died a physical death being torn apart by dinosaurs, they found that they were trapped on Earth. Although they were already trapped and hadn't realized it, they blamed the Lemurians for this and made many judgments against the Will. Lemurians also made many judgments here about Spirit and My Light.

This situation led to further misunderstandings, and without the understandings needed, great fear arose. Feeling that only the Will energy could be trusted was a problem for Lemuria. Their Spirits weren't allowed to be present, and I was banished by the Lemurians who blamed Me for their plight. Without help from Spirit, the Lemurians became more and more frightened. They had no weapons or means to combat something as immense as the dinosaurs on their own.

The dinosaurs destroyed Lemuria's beautiful vegetation. Many Lemurians moved as far away from the dinosaurs as they could and went underground to protect themselves. By the time that the Lemurians were living underground and dinosaurs were destroying everything on the surface, their Wills were very undermined again. Pressured and threatened by the dinosaurs, the mental capabilities of many Lemurians began to seriously deteriorate. Living in this constant survival threat, they became savage in many of the ways the base nature of man has so often been pictured to be, and became like early humans, or cavemen, that modern science discovered later.

Some, Lemurians, however, remained more intact than others. They had some receptivity to Spirit and were able to trust enough to be shown the way to escape from Lemuria. I gave them a reed boat design that could withstand turbulent water. They managed to build these boats and leave Lemuria in search of other places to live.

Some of the Indians of the Western United States and into Central and South America, many of the Polynesians and some Hawaiians are descendants of people who fled Lemuria in this way. They all have legends about this, and their legends are accurate according to what they themselves experienced. If there is disagreement among these legends, it is because the small bands of people had somewhat different experiences. But, they did escape Lemuria, and then Lemuria sank and took most of the dinosaurs with it.

Even though it has been a long time, these past experiences are not cleared yet. The understandings needed about Pangea and Lemuria are many. Many who went to the polarity of Atlantis made judgments against the Will as Lemuria was going down. If you had these experiences, you will be able to feel them in your own consciousness when you are ready to heal them. Seeing the understandings is only part of it though; the feelings need to be brought forward into the Spirit's consciousness, as well. Connecting to your own experience here can trigger the release of the feelings. Allow the feelings without judging them to be the permanent state of affairs. Freeing the feelings can give you understandings that can, in turn, allow release of the judgments.

ATLANTIS

Atlantis began to flourish as a civilization toward the end of Lemuria's time. Atlantis was a huge continent, most of which is now under the Atlantic Ocean. It was a brilliant manifestation of Spirit energy, unfettered by any of what they viewed as limitations from the Will. A popularly held image is that Atlantis was the highest civilization ever to exist on the Earth. While many hold fond memories, or think they do, of Atlantis, most of the people holding these memories also have a strong affinity to the polarity of the Spirit.

The Atlantean civilization was peopled by those who had had serious misgivings about free Will from the beginning and also by many who had become disenchanted with the polarization to the Will in Lemuria. Atlanteans wanted unfettered expansion on all levels. They wanted to elevate all manifestations of the Spirit and use and control the intuitive, feeling Will.

The Atlantean approach to life showed this polarization in all of its aspects. While communication in Lemuria was largely body language and empathic communication of feelings, communication in Atlantis was verbally articulate and developed expressions of complex thought patterns and visions that often flashed back and forth, quickly and telepathically. They also had many clear and detailed inner visions. Many in Atlantis developed the power of their mind to the point where they could focus thoughts and visions into crystals and store them there for their own later use or for presentation to groups of people. They could influence and control others, and they could also heal or harm with their powers.

Music in Atlantis consisted mainly of intricate, melodic patterns woven with voices and accompanied by stringed instruments that were also melodic. Music in Lemuria emphasized drums and rhythm. The buildings of Lemuria were earthen, while Atlanteans built refined, palatial structures of highly-polished stone. Murals, mosaics, sculptures, weavings, pottery, jewelry and all other art and artisan contributions to everyday life were highly refined examples of the visionary brilliance in Atlantis. Glassware and the carving of stones and gemstones became highly developed arts. Atlanteans felt it was important to study, consider, refine and develop the expression of the creative impulse. Lemurians, on the other hand, built, created and expressed with the feelings and spontaneity they valued so highly.

While travel for Lemurians consisted of walking, running, swinging through the trees with the help of branches and vines, leaping, soaring and teleporting rather great distances at a time, Atlanteans did not consider this to be dignified enough for them. They built some roads and stately vehicles, had processions and regulated individual everyday travel so that it was orderly. Atlantis had everyday, individualized means of conveyance that could be somewhat described as basket-like. These could move by hovering above the ground and followed guide lines that had the appearance of narrow roads. They also had majestic ships that could travel on the seas and in the air. Many Atlanteans traveled rather extensively and some had the means to own their own air and sea ships.

Atlantis developed an extensive technology. Repetitious tasks, and everything that seemed like drudgery to Atlanteans, received help from technology. Whatever was unsuitable for Atlanteans to do and unadaptable to their technology, was done by the sub-citizens of Atlantis. Sub-citizens consisted of beings still trapped in forms that limited them, Lemurians who had been brought there by Atlanteans to escape the dinosaurs, but were not "like" the Atlanteans, and later, some of the "strange" peoples from Pangea that Atlanteans had found in remote parts of the world. Atlanteans used these beings like slaves, and some abused them.

Many Atlanteans tried to ignore the humanness in these beings and rationalized the right of Atlantis to use them however they wanted to. Some Atlanteans wanted to ignore the uncomfortable imbalance with the Will these beings presented, and some wanted to help these beings evolve into the kind of consciousness they had.

Lemuria had not developed any technology, but they felt it was fun to do most of the things they did because they did them together and because they loved doing things with their physical body. The Atlantean point of view saw technology as an improvement on the Will and a relief from having to do much with their physical body. The power source for Atlantean technology was an energy they had learned to focus, store and project with the help of crystals. The development of technology in Atlantis was largely a compensation for power lost by denying the Will. Many more people, at that time, had a desire to provide themselves with a technological substitute for the powers of the Will, than had desire to understand and evolve the emotional quality of the Will.

At that time, the Spirits did not take responsibility for their own part in the imbalance. Instead, almost universally, the Spirits decided they wanted little to do with the Will, and that what Will remained with them needed to be controlled so that there were no repeats of what they judged had happened earlier. Since most Atlanteans saw the earlier problems of imbalance as something that could be solved if the Spirit was in control, the Spirit polarity in Atlantis began to emphasize regulation, discipline and orderly procedure in place of spontaneity and doing what they felt like doing.

At first, the Will in Atlantis went along with this and did not object or try to influence the Spirit. The Will really did fear that it had not done well in the past. Experience in Lemuria had seemed to show that the Will could not succeed on its own, and so, should find a way to agree with the Spirit and try to do what the Spirit wanted done. The Will in Atlantis was holding a large and unexpressed emotional charge around the question of what its appropriate role with the Spirit was supposed to be. The Spirit in Atlantis sought to educate the Will, and thus, train the Will to properly serve the Spirit. The Will in Atlantis tried to go along with this and be obedient to the Spirit.

All aspects of Atlantean society reflected these attitudes toward the Spirit and the Will. Religion and education were not separate in Atlantis. All Atlanteans who were capable of receiving an education, received an extensive education in the temples. Teachers in Atlantis were also students, in that they studied for their entire lives. Many realms of study were pursued in depth in Atlantis that have not received wide acceptance today as valid areas of study, and some are not consciously remembered at all. The sub-citizens, however, were taught only what Atlanteans decided they needed to know.

Atlantis developed the perceptive or "extra-sensory" powers extensively, and this study opened realms not perceived by many today. Everything Atlantis developed was inspired and guided by these expanded perceptions and the understandings received through them. Even though Atlantis had a scientific orientation, no one at that time considered these perceptions to be unscientific. The Atlanteans' ability to apply inspiration to everyday life also increased the credibility of receiving information from other realities, other kinds of beings and even from other planets.

The Atlantean civilization appeared to be fabulously successful for a long time. Everything they envisioned, and decided to try, came into manifestation and worked for them. Atlanteans saw this as evidence that they had true understanding. Their touch at that time was so infused with their Spirit light that it enlivened in ways seldom experienced now on Earth, and yet, most of the Will in Atlantis was not being touched by the Spirit at all and was hardly vibrating.

Atlanteans did not believe they were judging the Will or seeing its role inaccurately, and they did not realize that they had any denials. They believed the Will was meant to serve them. There were some reflections of their denials in Atlantis, but rather than accepting these, Atlanteans explained them away and, also, tried to ignore them. Atlanteans were holding beliefs and judgments about reality, and also, being proud of their accomplishments, mistook these judgments for reality.

One reflection which Atlanteans found to be uncomfortable and difficult to accept, and was, therefore, misunderstood was Lemuria. Many Atlanteans saw the overwhelming emotion held by the Will as the reason why Lemurians could not solve their problems. Believing the solution was to control the emotions of the Will, this belief powered much of the Atlantean approach. Total understanding and full acceptance was not fully present in the consciousness and, so, what has taken place has been necessary, and yet, it was, for the most part, a terrible experience for the Will in the last days of Pangea and Lemuria and in Atlantis. Rather than denying the experience of the Will further, there is much that can be learned about balance by studying these experiences of the past and releasing the feelings still held from them.

The Lemurians had developed the magnetic Will energy to a place of great power. By nature, magnetic Will energy is meant to attract the Spirit to it. Since the Will in Lemuria feared it was unaccepted by the Spirit and responded by reacting against it, Lemurians were unable to draw to themselves the increase in Spiritual presence necessary to guide the increased magnetic energy. Instead, the Lemurians drew to themselves, without realizing how they were doing it, not only manifestations of denied Spirit, but also a light that denied them. One of the forms this took was the dinosaurs, whose forms embodied every aspect of the judgments against Spirit that so many Lemurians held. Seeing this experience, many Spirits saw it as dangerous for the Will to vibrate unless the Spirit filled that space with light. Judging they were not going to be allowed to fill the space further fueled many Spirits in Atlantis to believe they had to make the Will be obedient to them.

This has to be understood individually, but some understandings can be given to help point the way. Many Lemurians had fear that the Spirit was an unloving, insensitive, domineering, controlling, overpowering, punishing monster that abandoned the Will right when the Will needed Spirit the most and had sent this upon them when they were doing their best to live on their own as they believed the Spirit wanted them to do. There was a firm belief in the Will that it was caught in a reality where the Spirit wouldn't help it, and that the Will was not supposed to ask for the Spirit's help or need it. Many in the Will-polarity felt that the Spirit had been, and still was, capable of hurting the Will by denying it and forcing experiences on it that were unpleasant and impossible for the Will to handle. Many even felt that Spirit was trying to kill it.

A secret fantasy of quite a few Lemurians was that if their situation became desperate enough, maybe the Spirit would realize it needed and loved the Will and would then dramatically rescue the Will and heal the split. This fantasy of hope was accompanied by a counterweight of fear that the Spirit would not help and would not come down into the murky realms where the Will was trapped. When I did not seem to help with Divine Intervention in the form that the Lemurians were seeking, some Lemurians finally appealed to the Atlanteans for help. Lemurians hoped that the Atlanteans would solve their problems for them, and yet, their judgments against the Spirit were also acted out there.

The Atlanteans were resistant to doing anything to help the Lemurians. They delayed for quite a while. When they finally did arrive on the scene, they were uncomfortable with the emotionality of the Lemurians. It was just what they sought to escape by living in Atlantis, and yet, the Atlanteans did decide to help. They wanted to help Lemuria as quickly and with as much detachment as they could, and leave as soon as possible. The Atlanteans decided to try out their crystal power by focusing it into the nesting grounds of the dinosaurs.

The Lemurians felt an instinctive objection to this which was disregarded by the Atlanteans as superstition and resistance to help. The Atlanteans offered to take to Atlantis any Lemurians who were willing to go. Many Lemurians felt this would be an unpleasant experience, and only some could detach from their homeland enough to go. The Atlanteans saw the Lemurians as overwhelmed by undirected emotion that lacked the vision and detachment necessary to solve their problems. They also saw it as necessary to take matters into their own hands as, in their view; nothing was going to be acceptable to the Lemurians. The Will in Lemuria felt denied by the Spirit once again and felt it could only watch powerlessly as a rather cold and detached Spirit dealt with the "failures" of the Will.

In denial of their own Wills, the Atlanteans were unable to see themselves as having any causal role here. They did not see their own involvement in how denied emotion was creating its own reflection in the dinosaurs. The focus of crystal power only temporarily set back the dinosaur population and directly resulted in volcanoes and earthquakes that, in the end, sank Lemuria. This was just what the intuitional Will in Lemuria had feared and was another experience that seemed to further prove the judgments against the Spirit. Some Lemurians also saw that their magnetic Will power had drawn exactly what they feared. They judged against themselves and their fear. This experience, without the understandings needed, led to a substantial increase in the polarization between Spirit and Will, and reinforced denial of the Will and its powers, even among many of those who had formerly believed in the Will or had viewed themselves as sympathetic toward the Will.

The Atlanteans did not admit that they had had anything to do with the sinking of Lemuria, but they did come back to Lemuria in its last days and offer again to take back to Atlantis any and all Lemurians who would agree to go. In Atlantis, these Lemurians received a mixed reception and, with few exceptions, were treated like sub-citizens. Many Atlanteans had not wanted to take in the Lemurians in the first place, and did not regard as valid any information that linked the sinking of Lemuria to the use of crystal power.

This experience of polarizing to the Spirit was necessary because the Spirit, at that time, did not understand the Will enough to balance with it. Without receptivity from the Spirit, the Will felt it had to wait. The accumulating charge in the Will during Lemurian times was causing many Wills to feel unable to do anything. This paralysis seemed to further the Atlantean theories that the Will could not be the determining factor. Most Atlanteans began scheduling their lives to substitute for the loss of direction from the Will. The Spirit's conceptualized vision pushed on the rest of the being to act. A common judgment reiterated, then, was that the Will holds the Spirit back and that the "lower nature" should not be allowed influence since, "the Spirit is willing, but the flesh is weak."

Atlantis went ahead, after Lemuria sank, and explored the rest of the world to see what was there. The many varied peoples and animals discovered in the world at that time both fascinated and disquieted them, but the Atlanteans chose to focus on their fascination and, for the most part, ignored their disquietude. On the Earth at that time were many scattered bands of people who had fled Pangea. These different groups had varying residual effects from the land of Pan, depending on their particular experiences and their point of view. Among these peoples, Atlanteans found groups of giants many feet tall, and even as tall as twenty-five feet, bands of dwarves, bands of little people as small as a foot tall and numerous others. I also want to say that some, whose men were only around 6 inches tall, fully grown, were able to hide successfully from the Atlanteans. Some still had forms that were a mixture of man and animal, such as satyrs, centaurs and mer-people. Some people still had gills. Some of these peoples had a highly-developed consciousness, and some had forms that severely limited the ability of their consciousness to be present or to express itself.

In studying these peoples, the Atlanteans tried to put many pieces of the picture together about the history on Earth up to that time, but everything was filtered through their own viewpoint. The vision of the Spirit in Atlantis was to bring together, under its direction, the scattered bands, and their scattered pictures of reality, into a cohesive, unified whole, but most of these differing beings did not want to align with the vision of Atlantis. Many of the people at that time felt alienated from everything except their own viewpoint, the Atlanteans included.

The Atlanteans did not know how to bring this diversity into willing alignment. And so, once again, the Will was blamed and judged as being in opposition to the Spirit. Undercurrents of frustration, fear and anger grew behind these judgments, and since the Atlanteans had left no avenue open to accept these feelings and bring them into loving alignment, they concluded that they had no recourse but to overpower these peoples. Objections voiced directly to the powers in Atlantis often resulted in imprisonment.

Their own denied feelings empowered the action they took. Atlantis resorted to a demonstration of the destructive power of their great crystal, hitting a settlement they feared, but thought they hated the most: a settlement of giants. They showed pictures of this destruction to the peoples who did not want to accept Atlantean domination, and feeling powerless against this force, most of these peoples gave in or appeared to give in. Atlantis, then, became the undisputed ruler of the world.

Understandings cannot come disconnected from experience. Understandings must come in a progression as experience creates a readiness to receive them. Many Spirits had received an overload in the beginning by trying to gain understandings without the necessary experience in which to anchor them. Many of these Spirits still continued trying to preach to their Wills, telling them how they should perform in relationship to the understandings the Spirit thought it had, but in actuality, were only conceived of by the Spirit at that time, and had need of Will and Body's experiences to grow to maturity. The Will was distrustful of Spirit because it was feeling overwhelmed by experiences that were much more complex and difficult than the Spirit's concepts had represented them to be. Instead of receiving the Will here, the Spirit was denying and maligning what Will and Body were experiencing.

In Atlantis, the Will was not opposed to the vision of the Spirit so much as to the ways the Atlanteans were going about implementing it. The Will had wanted to have its feelings accepted. Then, it might have felt more ready to receive the Spirit. The Spirit was still feeling more than uncertain about wanting to have much at all to do with the Will. The Spirit wanted the Will to accept it on its own terms, and told itself it might, then, be more receptive to what the Will wanted to say.

As time went on, Atlantis entered what could be called its middle period. The Will reached the place where it could no longer obediently hold its growing charge. Now, whether the Will understood itself or not, it began to stir. Feelings and desires that Atlanteans thought they had disciplined, refined and evolved out of themselves began to stir again. When the suppressed Will in Atalantis began to move, it was under the heavy weight of judgments that Atlanteans were holding there. Many Atlanteans began to express aspects of themselves that they had not been expressing earlier, especially sexually. Many unexpressed emotions and judgments were channeled into this sexual expression.

Conflict arose again within the self, concerning morals and correct spiritual approach. Disagreements between individuals increased. Some people began to express more of what they were really feeling. In others, the Will began to have more influence over the way they approached their lives. Neat schedules and orderly procedures began to break down as people began to do a little more of what they felt like doing, rather than just what they had been told they were supposed to do. Many in Atlantis who began to do what they wanted to do made up reasons why they were supposed to do it or why they had to do it. The lack of alignment in Atlantis between the Spirit and the Will made them feel that what they wanted to do was something other than what they were supposed to do. The conflict between duty and desire made room for an increase in guilt that they should be feeling and doing differently than they were.

The Spiritual presence in Atlantis had deeply denied fears about what had happened in Lemuria which they did not recognize as fear of the Will. They still believed that the Will was not willing to align with the Spirit. They still believed that control of the Will was essential and that if the Will got out of control, it would destroy everything. Because of its overwhelming initial experience of entry into Earth, the Spirit believed it must deny the Will in order to not be denied itself. In Atlantis this meant that the Will was to express only in the ways the Spirit allowed.

The Will felt it was being told again that only certain aspects of itself were acceptable to the Spirit. The Spirit seemed to confirm this by not touching the Will with its light in these judged against areas. The Will, however, had the feelings that it had about its experience on Earth, whether the Spirit accepted them or not. The Spirit denied these feelings because they did not feel good to it, and tried to avoid these feelings in the Will by not allowing them to move and express. The Spirit believed that if it did not allow the Will to move freely, the Will could not move into the areas that had been so unpleasant for the Spirit. The Will, then, had tremendous obstacles to being able to clear what it was holding.

When the Will began to stir again in Atlantis, the Atlanteans responded with more controls, regulations, disciplines and pressure to conform. When the Will in Atlantis could not continue to hold its growing charge, it still tried to move in any way it could. When the Will cannot gain release, at least some of the Will's overload is held in the physical Body. When the physical Body could no longer hold what the emotions were not being allowed to express, the physical Body tried to move it in a physical way. Discord, violence, sexual expression and illness increasingly became Body's avenues of expression for attempting to clear itself.

As denial of the Will went on, the health of Atlanteans began to break down. Instead of allowing illness to express and tell its story of imbalance so that balance could be found, the Atlanteans applied their sound, light and other therapies for healing Body with greater fervor to combat this growing "sabotage" of Will and Body. Medical treatment and treatment of insanity took a punitive and suppressive approach toward the Body and the emotions. In some cases, Atlanteans even resorted to surgery.

Although, when problems have advanced too far and no other means of healing are known or understood, surgery, and other drastic measures may be necessary, the concept of cutting out an ailing part of the Body and throwing it away is not really more advanced than human sacrifice. Both of these approaches believe a part can be sacrificed for the good of the whole. In both cases, understanding can bring balance before such drastic measures are needed.

If an accident is manifested or a part of the Body is ailing, then something is impeding its ability to receive loving light. What the Spirit denied in Atlantis, it did not nourish with its light. When the Spirit blocked the clearance that Will and Body needed, both the Will and the Body began to feel desperate. This desperation carried Atlantis into its third and final period.

The more the Spirit tried to control the Will, the more the Will's held charge grew from fear, anger and sadness into terror, rage and heartbreak. The Will was feeling denied, overwhelmed and compressed beyond its ability to endure. The Will feared it could not clear itself if the Spirit would not allow it, and it could not continue feeling what it was feeling with no relief. The Will was not being allowed to vibrate itself. It felt that the Spirit was killing it and, in truth, the Spirit really was doing this to its own Will.

The Will cannot live unless it vibrates. When the Will vibrates, it opens space. When space is opened, something has to fill it. If the Spirit does not fill the space with loving light, then denial fills the space. When something in the Will is completely ignored, that area of the Will receives, in effect, nothing. When this happens, the experience of the Will is the experience of opening to receive nothing or, even worse, opening and receiving unlovingness. No amount of pressure, force or imposed procedure is going to fill this space in the right way. When the Will cannot move, density increases until there is no vibration, which is death. The Will has to be free to move, and the Spirit has to fill this space with Loving Light.

In the final period of Atlantis, the desperation of the Will manifested itself in any way that it could. The old charge of the Will was trying frantically to clear itself. The more it tried to move, the harder it was hit with denial. Every attempt it made to release itself that was not met by acceptance from the Spirit, was met with more denials in the form of controls and reprisals by those still attempting to cling to the belief that control of the Will was absolutely necessary. These people continued to hold their judgments against the Will and viewed the action of the Will as further proof that the Will was denying of and in opposition to the Spirit.

The social manifestations of the Will's desperation were many. Increased pressure on the Will caused the Wills of some to break through the controls of the Spirit and express in an "out of control" manner. Often, the disconnect between the Will and the Spirit was so severe that it was as though a stranger had taken over the normally, Spirit-oriented personality. Many could not remember what they had done during these outbreaks. The lack of alignment between the Will and the Spirit was also acted out on a larger scale in society. Wars broke out in outlying regions. Disorder, civil disobedience and crime increased in Atlantis itself.

Denial in Atlantis had placed so much of its energy field outside of loving acceptance, that loving essence that was denied and, thus, placed outside of love, became mixed in with unconditional denial. Denial that had no loving essence was already present in Atlantis. Now, it began to find more ways to manifest its presence. The Will did not want this, and when it felt itself in the presence of this denial, it felt terrified. Some Will essence leapt toward the Spirit, trying to gain its attention any way it could. Even so, the Will still could not express all the emotion it felt regarding its situation, and, so, it didn't find out that, by doing this, it could have been able to let go of the denial mixed in with it that did not want love and light.

The people of Atlantis had little to no awareness of the role being played by denial. Instead of accepting, and growing to understand, the Will's attempts to clear itself of denial it had received, many Atlanteans still attempted to deny the Will further. Society enforced this viewpoint of denying the Will by killing, torturing, jailing, drugging, confining to hospitals and otherwise penalizing many in Atlantis who were without conscious understanding of what they were doing, but were trying to clear their Wills. The desperate action that some Wills were taking in the final period of Atlantis was seen by many Spirits as further proof that drastic reprisals aimed at controlling the Will were more necessary than ever. Repression was increased, and a deaf ear was turned to the viewpoint of the Will. The fear of the Will that its attempts to clear itself would only result in further denial was manifesting itself in reality.

Based on what the Spirits in power positions in Atlantis were still seeing as the resistance, opposition and limitations of the Will toward the Spirit, a decision was made to rev-up the Great Crystal in an attempt to display such a force of power that dissidence and rebellion would be quelled. The Atlanteans who did this over-amped the Great Crystal with more energy than it could hold; much of it filled with an intent to destroy the Will. This was another reenactment of Spirit attempting to rev-up and expand without regard for the Will's willingness or ability to receive and ground this energy. As a result, the discharge of this excessive energy manifested as an undirected force that did extensive damage and resulted in earthquakes that, ultimately, sank Atlantis.

Toward the end of Atlantis, a number of people who had more openness, and really were seeking more balance with the Mother energy, decided they had to leave Atlantis. They planned

107

to leave in boats, and decided that they would have to be built in secret. By the time they were ready to leave, earthquakes were already causing dangerous rip-tides and tidal waves, but they were able to receive some guidance from Me and succeeded in finding another place to live. Many of them became the original people of the Eastern and Central American cultures.

Even as their land was sinking, many Atlanteans, however, were still denying that there was any connection between their beliefs, the way they implemented their beliefs and the problems manifesting in Atlantis. Instead, these Atlanteans further intensified the split between the Spirit and the Will by continuing to claim that their beliefs were correct and that the reason their belief system was not successful was because the Will was at fault. Some of these people escaped from their sinking land and went to what had been outlying regions of Atlantis to try to continue their way of life. Egypt, Persia and a number of other places that made sudden leaps in their civilization did so because Atlanteans came to live there.

Since physical death had become a reality on Earth, many more people died in Atlantis as earthquakes and sinkings swept the land, and they did not have the means to escape. A number of them died in confinement and imprisonment. The fear of the Spirit that the Will would deny it, and the fear of the Will that the Spirit would deny it, was manifesting in reality. The judgments, made again by everyone in the last days of Atlantis were against both the Spirit and the Will. Some leaned toward one polarity and some toward the other. Reality is that one polarity cannot be denied without denial of the other polarity also taking place. Most of these judgments are still present, and they have lessened the brilliance of present society. Even so, over and over, many Atlanteans have still wanted to try their approach again, and have continued to hold the dream of restoring the brilliance they once knew in Atlantis. Much of "modern" society has been primarily Atlantean in outlook. Those discriminated against in these societies have, for the most part, been the more Will-oriented and have had a Lemurian approach or have leaned in this direction. The role played by denial has still been largely ignored.

So many judgments have been made during the course of experiences on Earth, and empowered to stay present by unreleased emotion, that these judgments cannot all be listed. The main focus of the judgments in Atlantis was that loss of control is very dangerous and that the expression of the Will brings chaos, that the Will must not be allowed to express because it is destructive, that the Will is, by nature, in opposition to the Spirit and must be disciplined, controlled and suppressed, that the information from the intuitional faculty of the Will cannot be trusted, that the Will's contribution to Creation is in conflict with the Spirit's vision, that the Will is the cause of death and that there is nothing the Spirit can do about this except rise above it and leave it behind and that Will and Body are meant to serve the Spirit, and are not meant to have a say in Creation, anyway.

The presence of Atlantean and Lemurian consciousness on Earth today can show you the judgments still held from those times. The vast wealth of information that could be brought forward from the past also cannot be done within the limitations of a book. These stories have brought forward some of the information that needs to be enlarged upon by individual memory. The process of clearing your own Will can allow it to tell its story.

DRUGS

I am now going to seem, perhaps, to diverge here and give some understandings on drugs. It is not really a divergence, however, since drugs have been used by people on Earth almost since the original loss of consciousness in Pangea. Since then, people have used drugs to increase the split between Spirit and Will, even to the extreme of dying to escape feelings and consciousness they haven't wanted to accept, and also, to try to heal the split and regain feelings and consciousness they have believed they lost.

Understandings are needed about drugs, including all of the currently popular, consciousness-altering drugs. The use of drugs is not being recommended by Me because there are numerous risks involved. In addition to the known risks, there are also unknown and, currently, unsuspected risks, including the risk that drugs can open your energy field to things you do not fully understand. While drugs can temporarily alleviate unbearable pain, it is necessary to protect the energy field of the person using drugs so that other influences cannot enter.

Drugs can alter your consciousness in ways that your usual, everyday level of vibration does not normally experience. These drugs can show you more that you can assimilate into your consciousness. In this way, some drugs can help show the way, but they are not the way, in that they cannot do it for you. You must still utilize the information to increase your own awareness and vibration. The use of these drugs is not helpful if the insights gained from them are not integrated into the person's normal state of consciousness. The person using drugs needs to know how they can help. Drugs are not help when they take the form of dependency or addiction. Then, you may have to reclaim your personal power from the drugs. This might even mean going over all of the steps you thought you were taking toward healing, again, without the drugs.

Drugs have often been used to override, disconnect from or rise above the Will and Body. Drugs are substances that can be difficult for the Body to eliminate, especially if the Will is undermined, and the Will of everyone on Earth today is undermined. The accumulation of drug residue can have a gradually increasing and deadening effect on Will and Body and can be noticed as reduced function and reduced sensitivity. The dosage of the drug must then be increased to produce a similar effect. This increases the residue, which calls for increased dosage once again. Given the accumulative effects of drugs, these drug induced impairments and losses can be gradual enough that they may not be noticed until, for many people, they are irreversible and, sooner or later, except in cases of people who would not be alive without certain medications, results in an earlier death than would have been likely, otherwise.

Drugs have, so far, shown themselves to be treacherous because of their ability to gain a hold on the ones using them. Any judgment held about drugs affects the experience of the ones using them. If someone believes he/she must have a drug, then he/she must have it. If belief is held that a drug is necessary to get high, or that pain can't be handled without drugs, then that will be the person's reality. Some of these beliefs are held at very deep levels and can require a considerable amount of deep movement to shift effectively.

Many people have had an uneasy, unsettled, empty feeling that they have tried to avoid in this and other ways. Some people have masked and avoided symptoms with drugs until the Body's problems have become extensive and serious. If surgery is required, even anesthesia for surgery will result in eventually having to accept both the pain of the surgery and the other levels of pain that that part of the Body accumulated from the denials it received and had to hold when the messages of its symptoms were not being accepted.

Drugs have a place like everything else. Sometimes relief from pain is necessary; sometimes expansion of consciousness is helped, but for many, drugs have declined into a habit pattern which is not helpful. Drugs have actually damaged many more people than they have helped. So, be careful with the use of drugs; all drugs.

If you want to recover your Will, drugs may not be what they seem to be. In more people than not, the relief, the upliftment, the increased consciousness, or whatever was originally sought, has, with habit and time, taken them where their conscious mind did not think it was going to go. Habitual, long-term drug use can become the decreased consciousness the drug-users were seeking to transcend when they began using the drugs. As your Will becomes free and more attuned, you probably will not want to use drugs, but nothing should be entirely ruled out. However, I will emphasize that drugs can be a treacherous path that can lead you into your own pit of denials whether you are ready or not, and whether you know how to handle this or not.

An understanding also needing mention is that people are not ultimately meant to decide about the use, or non-use, of drugs for one another. Once again, denials have played a large role in this intimidating form. When some people judged drugs to be damaging, they may have been accurate as far as their knowledge went, but the form of a judgment is not useful. More than the drugs, it is the consciousness using them that is the determining factor. Drugs cannot be used to permanently further your own denials or to avoid what has seemed too unpleasant or too overwhelming, without having to recover this denied essence later.

Healing the whole self includes bringing consciousness and the healing presence of Loving Light into all places of pain. You need to let yourself be aware of what you are doing and why you are doing it, and be willing to accept, as soon as you can, anything that drugs have been helping you escape, such as intense pain or grief. Nothing is left unfelt when you are completely present with yourself. Any space in which you were unconscious holds feelings that need to be accepted when you can. This is not to say that you are always going to be in pain if you don't shut anything out. Unconsciousness is the response of not being able, or not being willing, to accept something when it is happening. Responsibility for disconnection and denial must be taken as soon as the Spirit involved is able to do it.

Spirit and Heart, as well as Will and Body, actually do remember the pain of surgery and everything else that has been experienced and remembers this, even from life to life. And so, at some point, everything will have to come forward to be cleared and given a place of acceptance. The loss of memory of recent past lives, and even distant existences in places such as Pan, Lemuria and Atlantis, is all based in denial. If you use drugs, use them with these understandings in mind and not to increase your own denials.

UNDERSTANDINGS ON DENIAL

Different kinds of Spirits like different kinds of situations and societies. There is no problem here if no force is used to make anyone live in any way that is not compatible with their own nature. Lemuria and Atlantis both had problems from the disconnect of Will and Spirit, but they also both had problems because all the different kinds of Spirits living in those societies could not approach life in just the same way. Minorities need a place in which they can freely do what they feel is the right thing for them. If this brings to mind fear that people will get out of control, you need to realize that you are carrying that judgment. Societies on Earth have been based in denial since the beginning, and people do not yet have the experience of society without denial.

Society actually can be based on an aligned Spirit and Will balancing in the Heart. Society on Earth is going to change in the next few years so that Spirit and Will can express freely from the Heart. Alignment of individuals will align society. This transformation is just as possible as transforming the entire Body with the consciousness. Anything you heal is a transformation; the definition of healing must be expanded to include returning yourself to your full consciousness by healing all the separations within yourself and between yourself and Me.

Because I am everywhere and everything, this separation has been said by many to be "simply illusion." In a sense, it is illusion, but the "illusion of separation" concept has been applied in two ways that I want to point out here. While one way has been to go to the extreme of insisting that there is no separation going on at all, in terms of the everyday experience of most people, separation has not felt like an illusion. Another way has been to take the idea of separation to the extreme of insisting that I am not present at all, that I am a remote God who doesn't care or look to Earth, or even that I don't exist. Many of these people have acted as though there has been a successful separation from origin and from whatever parts of the self have not been accepted. Both of these views have some truth in them, and also some denial. I can be shut out, and that is what most people on Earth have had in common; a feeling that I shut them out because I didn't like them or that they shut Me out because they didn't like Me, or both.

I have differentiated My Energy into many forms. Different Spirits accept Me in different ways, in different forms and in varying intensities. There is no problem with this, unless there are denials. People can fool themselves when denials are present, and I say there is hidden denial here, in most cases. The hidden denials here are of self and of Me. When the self is denied, I am denied. Some Spirits who have denied My presence on Earth are really not wanting Me to be there and have created an illusion they have been insisting is reality. Some Spirits avoid My presence so they can avoid their feelings about Me. Some convert all of their feelings about Me into what they call worship, and others "worship" just in case they might go to Hell otherwise. Some Spirits, who say they recognize Me in everything, have denied some of their own feelings about Form.

Everything is not the same or it would not have differentiated into so many various forms. Form is not something to be denied. This is among the many ways Spirits have denied their own feelings of anger, fear and other feelings they have toward Me, toward Creation or both. I want to point out that all differentiation of energy into Form has been termed an illusion by some. The ones saying this do not fully understand Form, and whether they realize it or not, have judged against Me. Two of these judgments are that I should not have manifested this Creation, and that, conversely, I have only created an illusion of having created anything, and that really, everything is still the same as it always was and, so, nothing ever changes. This is also, then, a judgment against experience. This is not something to take lightly here. Judging against My Creation and the experiencing of it is judging against My evolutionary process and your own, too, for that matter. Buried here are often feelings of not liking Creation the way it is, and rather than notice this and acknowledge that they don't understand it, it has been easier to judge against it. If you hold this judgment, this will be your perspective. Rejection of My

Creation is possible, but this, then, will be your own experience and not the experience of My Creation as a whole.

Many Spirits have made these judgments without realizing what they were really doing. Some have believed the views of others to be the reality, and some avoid their feelings of lack of acceptance for themselves, others and Creation by hiding their feelings behind the belief that "all is illusion." I wanted to comment on this because it is a confusion that has been very widespread on Earth. Many who have claimed they accept Me, have accepted Me only as Light and have not accepted My Forms. Others who have been caught up in the world of Form have claimed that they do not need My Presence as Light because they accept Me as Form.

I am both Light and Form, and Spirits need to accept Me as both. The split toward Me is part of the separation illusion on Earth. It is a very real separation, too, since almost no one on Earth is now able to speed up the physical Body until it becomes Light. Some Spirits think the loss of this ability is not a problem because they have been believing that physicality means density, and so it is not appropriate for the physical body to become light. This is another judgment, and not true understanding. All energy is meant to be free. Your physical body is a part of you and is only meant to be physical if it wants to be. Many have made assumptions here that because Body is physical, it wants to be. This would be true if everything were aligned. As you clear your energy, your physical body is going to become more and more light-filled, and you are going to regain lost abilities. This is going to proceed at the speed at which your layers of conditioning can truly open to align with and receive My Loving Light. My words here are not meant to sound like pressure. You can take your own path, and I can put you in your right place where you can progress at the speed that feels right to you.

Some Spirits who have said that it makes no difference how they receive Me, really do have feelings here that do not want to see Me being limited to the present reality on Earth. These Spirits would also like Me to be present with them in ways they can hear in words, see as light, feel as the presence of unconditional love and experience as the power to transform themselves and their lives on Earth. This desire is not a fantasy that only takes place after death; it is real and is something that can happen now. This is something that you can find within your own being if you want it. This is not something that is too difficult to do either, but it may involve more than you at first thought that it would. The journey

114

to your full consciousness and your full awareness of Me is going to be full of adventure for you and is the most exciting journey you could take. While it is true that everything you experience is a part of your journey; some routes are more direct than others, some routes more painful than others.

Some have said that it is not possible to be out of alignment, anyway. This is another way in which Spirits have been avoiding their feelings of fear and panic held in a state of denial. Lack of alignment with the self and with Me is the actual state of many on Earth. The illusion that nothing can be done to make it different is another judgment that has been a way to explain away things that they have felt would, otherwise, be too overwhelming to accept. This is called denial.

When you feel that you are not able to accept what is happening to you because it is too overwhelming, and you, instead, tell yourself that it is not really happening, the way is opened for judgments, misunderstandings, illusions, emotional blockage and everything else that is needing to be cleared on Earth right now. Denial is what is happening when you cannot accept your own experience. This denial has been increasing on Earth over time.

In the beginning, denial was not thought to be much. It began with denial of some feelings that were not experienced to be as pleasant as other feelings. When these feelings came up, they began to be avoided and not accepted or expressed. In the beginning, this was not even thought to be denial. The feelings were not thoroughly understood then, and many thought that they could be accepted or not in the same way that other experiences could be accepted or not. Feelings, however, are not something exterior like other experiences. They are also not something that has just been made up by the mind, and so, cannot just be rearranged by the mind. Feelings are the counterpoint to the mind and a real part of the self. Many Spirits were confused on this issue and rejected feelings they did not like. This was rejecting a part of themselves. Rejecting a part of the self is not possible without reclaiming it later.

The increase in denial has mainly taken place in this way: Rather than rejecting experiences that did not feel good, many Spirits rejected their feelings about these experiences instead. In the beginning, before the response of the Will was warped by denial, the feelings were only responsive. They were not causing an experience to be unpleasant. Feelings are the Will's response to what it is experiencing. When they did not like their Will's response, many Spirits overrode their Wills and denied the validity of their Will's response. Among all the Spirits, the entire spectrum exists from no denial to complete denial. Early experience overwhelmed many Spirits because they were not heeding their Wills and removing themselves from experiences that they did not like.

There was another misunderstanding present here among many Spirits, and that was that they should ignore their own limitations and experience everything because I did. The ones trying this had another misunderstanding about right time. They were not ready. Some denied this by saying, "Time is an illusion."

The accumulation of experience is not an illusion, and that amounts to time. There is a pattern of denial here. Some have had this pattern because of confusion and misunderstandings, and some because they thought that they could deny the reality of their own experiences in this way. Some have denied ever making judgments. Some have denied that they have any misunderstandings, and some have denied that death is their intent. Once again, intent is the determining factor, and some Spirits have even been denying what their intent really is.

Blockages in the way of My presence can appear to have shut Me out, and as My Light can be reduced to almost nothing, and, sometimes, to nothing, I can appear to not be present. I am, in fact, no longer present in some cases where I have decided to put this essence outside of My Light. I am, however, still present in a state of denial in some very dense places. By not recognizing Light in such dense forms, some Spirits have convinced themselves that they have gotten away from Me. Others have convinced themselves that they are with Me because they recognize everything as a form of Light.

If your intention is to end your denial, you can end it once you realize that you have it and begin to recognize what your denials are. Since denial is so extensive on Earth right now, I need to point this out: When your denials are effective, you do not realize you have them. You are convinced that your denials are reality. Reality is that once you connect to some of your denials, you will find it easier to connect to the rest of them.

Denial on Earth needs to be cleared. Reality is going to change soon in such a way as to make the retention of denial impossible if you are going to stay on Earth. If you are not ready to end your

116

denials, you can continue them on another planet. A planet has the right to say who can live on it. Earth has chosen to have denial cleared and wants to return to its original vision of itself. This is why no one can remain on Earth and hold denial. I already see many Spirits who do not want to remain on Earth. Since I do not want Spirits to blame Me for removing them from Earth, I want all of you who feel ready to take responsibility for yourselves to decide if Earth is for you or not. Remaining on Earth means accepting the full self completely, clarifying intent to end personal denial and find balance in your Heart and being aligned with the Earth itself.

Instead of fastening on the idea that you must heal everything immediately, you need to start with yourself by making an unconditional acceptance of how it really feels to be you, and accept those feelings. You need to have a completely committed intent to end denial and heal all of the separations that your denials have created.

The Spirit must have acceptance for its lack of experience in Manifestation, and the Will must have acceptance for its emotional response to this. Spirit and Will must accept Themselves and Each Other here; then Heart and Body can receive the balanced energy They need. Suffering is the path of having experiences that you do not really want to have. I have not required suffering in order to come to Me. I have not required Spirits to test themselves in this way. I have not asked anyone to find out if courage is sufficient to go past fear. These are all misunderstandings of Me.

When I describe Original Cause, you will be able to see how all the various images of Me came to be. Suffice it to say for now, that I am a living, evolving God, and all the held images of Me are frozen pictures. Even the ones saying that they do not worship an image of Me are holding limits of one sort or another. For example, some believe that I am a human-like Father in Heaven, and some believe that I am so far beyond humans that I do not even speak to them anymore. Some believe that I am terrible, angry and judgmental while some believe I am impersonal and have no feelings at all. Some believe I watch everything they do, and some believe I never look at Earth. I could go on and on, but I believe that these examples will suffice to show you the understanding I want to impart. All of this is imagery and not the total picture of Me. Original Cause can help you to see how all of these pieces can fit together and be healed.

You need to heal yourself enough with what I am giving you now to be able to accept more. I also want to say that this channeling is clear, accurate, what I intend to say and from Me, which is not to say that you cannot question. If you feel doubts and fears within yourself, accept them, and let them find their right place in your process. Allow yourself the freedom to question, doubt and search within yourself until you feel for yourself what is true for you.

In summary, I want to point out that having experiences you cannot fully accept, along with the accompanying pain and denial, has not been increasing the presence of Loving Light within you. I also want to make you aware that, for all practical purposes, it is possible to take yourself out of existence in this way. Another understanding needed here is that denial does not generally result if you do not have an experience until you are ready for it. Since you cannot escape from what has happened already, you need to take responsibility for it, clear it and gain the understandings needed. In this way, you can learn how not to have to suffer from pain, fear or denial because you won't be creating it.

The question of the past has been raised by many who have said that the past is over, so forget it. Usually these people are referring to unpleasantness that they perceive as having occurred in the past, however, the idea that the past is past, as though it is somehow disconnected from the present, and so, does not influence it, is not true understanding. If it was really "over," it would not be affecting the present, and history would not be repeating itself. No matter how it may look at first, lack of understanding the past does not create beneficial change in the present, or the future. The past is part of a continuum which is not unchangeable. The past is a reservoir of wisdom available to the present. If what has not been liked about the past is not fully understood and utilized as a source of wisdom, even though it may change form somewhat, it will repeat in some form until it is accepted and understood. Acceptance brings Loving Light, which is what is needed for something to be able to change. Studying the past for what can be learned actually allows the present to become more free and more creative, more abundant and more open to change. Accepting, understanding and freeing what's been held in the past can change the present, and since the present is creating the future, it affects the future, too.

The past two hundred years or so in America have much to teach that has been largely denied and ignored. The people originally living in America had preserved everything so that the continent had everything to offer when America was "discovered." Their vast wisdom about how to live on this continent was disregarded, disrespected, even buried, trampled over and largely lost, so that most people have only scanty information about the past here.

The indigenous people who met the first explorers denied some of their true feelings in favor of ideas about what they should do. Denied because they did not like to feel them, these deep and mostly lost feelings had manifested as an outer reflection that brought to them their Karmic involvement in what happened. These old denials, drawn to the American Continent, were already affecting the "Old World," and have now affected the entire world, even if only remotely through the pollution and other side effects their presence has caused. Painful as it has been, and is, these denials need to be seen and understood for what they are.

These same beings have incarnated into America for several lives and have, each time, worked to further their denial of true feelings and of the Earth, itself. Denial has even been going on where you may think there has been acceptance. If you study this, rather than accepting it as it appears, you can see what I mean. For example, those who conceived the Constitution of the United States were intending to create freedom for themselves only.

Form has received so much denial that it can appear to misrepresent itself. For example, what has been represented as "the expansion necessary to life" has actually been the expansion of denial, compression and death. Seeing these denials personified as others and not understanding it, many have thought that this reflection was proving their judgments to be right. These are the kinds of experiences that do not need to keep happening if the needed understandings are gained.

Technology has been developed that can actually control and kill the Earth and everybody on it. I do not want to allow this to happen. Denial of fear and terror, in their many forms, and the accompanying old judgments, or subconscious imprints, has been causing this. These denials have their roots in Original Cause and were present in the first re-enactments on Earth, in the Land of Pan. Although the form has been changing, people have been re-enacting their Original Cause over and over because they have not had the understandings needed. I see that enough experience has been had now, and that many people are ready to heal what their original misunderstandings have brought to them.

Since the feelings give the Spirit the information needed to gain the understandings, denial of feelings is an effective way to short-circuit Spirit also. Many people have tried to deny this problem by saying that it isn't possible for Spirit to have any problems, but I want to say that it is entirely possible. It is even possible for a Spirit to decide it does not want to exist, but those who have made this choice should not be allowed to take others with them.

Since I do not want any of My Spirits to go down the path of denial any longer without knowing what they are doing so that they can make a choice, I have decided that intervention is necessary. I am offering the understandings needed and taking the actions necessary to straighten things out on Earth. Part of this action is taking the form of removing Spirits from Earth and putting them in their right place. This needs to be accepted by the ones remaining on Earth. I have tried to do this before, and each time, the ones remaining have drawn back to Earth the ones removed.

Acceptance of true feelings opens the space for Me to put Spirits in their right place. True feelings and right place must be accepted on Earth now. It can be seen that many things are not in their right place on Earth. True feelings must be accepted in order for things to go to their right place. Think about this, and see how it works for you in your own life. Denial cannot see what is really happening and cannot feel it, either. Things can then be out of place, and you do not let yourself recognize it or express yourself in the ways that would allow things to be in their right place in relationship to you.

Right place is tied in with loving acceptance also. Loving acceptance means that everything has a right to be in the place that is right for it. Denial of right place has allowed everything to mix together on Earth. In some cases, guilt has played a large role here, but so, also, has bad intent. It is true that loving acceptance does not deny anything, and yet, there was hidden denial here, even though many loving Spirits thought that there was not. Guilt has confused many into thinking that guilt is love. Love, however, does not involve self-denial and guilt always does. When Spirits have pressured themselves to accept other Spirits and experiences that they did not like, true feelings were denied there. These feelings were usually judged to be unloving. When you feel pressured by guilt, go to a private place and give expression to the emotions being triggered.

Denial opens space for denial Spirits to operate. If you have no denial, you have no denial Spirits around you to reflect your denials to you. Without denial, you are no longer right place for them. Expression of true feelings is going to make these things increasingly clear to you. There is dread on Earth of having things come out in the open. Denial has been the way many have avoided their dread, fear and even panic. This dread of seeing things as they are also has deep roots in Original Cause, but seeing things as they are is better, in the long run, than pretending that things are otherwise. It may be a great relief from the pressure of constantly pretending and trying to keep up appearances. Expression of true feelings can also create the movement needed to bring changes you can really like.

Spirits need to be ready for the experiences they have. Emotions are not to be denied in favor of the experiences that are triggering them. This is how many Spirits got themselves overwhelmed to the point where they felt they had to deny. Denial is now so much a part of everyone and everything that almost no one realizes they are doing it, and those who do, often realize it only later.

In Pan, many Spirits felt overwhelmed by the reality they saw before them. There were so many fast form changes that nothing seemed stable. These Spirits felt that they could not leave Earth. They felt they had no place else to go and no place else they wanted to go. These Spirits could not make the ones upsetting them leave Earth because of their confusions about loving acceptance. They, then, felt they had no way to go other than denial. Some denied the reality in front of them, and some denied their feelings about the reality in front of them. In increasing their denials, these Spirits did not realize the role their own denials were already playing. Denial compounded the problem it attempted to solve by allowing the situation to get much more out of hand than it would have otherwise, but at the time it seemed the only possible way to go.

Experience is still overwhelming many on Earth today. Many still feel that the situation has gotten so out of hand that they can't do anything but deny it. Many have been holding everything they feel about the world in general in denial, trying to live their lives as best they can, yet this is no longer the way they want their lives to be. Those who think that life on Earth, at present, is good, have lost their vision of how life could be and of how life is meant to be. Denial in your personal life has been enabling you to avoid what would otherwise make your life unpleasant and frightening.

In short, many feel they have been pushed to the wall on Earth. The denial now has to move; this is the only out available. The recognition and ending of denial is going to open the way for reclamation of power. Individual power is lost when parts of the self are placed in denial. Overpowering has taken place because of denial. When denial ends, overpowering will also end.

FORM AND GRAVEN IMAGES

The idea that everything is One is an accurate understanding, and yet, differentiation and delineation are necessary in order to experience this Oneness in Manifestation. Form has many things to teach, as does experience. There have been many misunderstandings about Form on Earth, and many understandings have been denied. Denial of the importance of Form has already imbalanced Form on Earth so seriously that it has not been able to fully express the consciousness within it. When this has happened, I have had to intervene to straighten this out enough that Form could stay in Manifestation.

Manifestation in Form must be respected, even by those who do not understand its purpose. The purpose of Manifestation is not fully understood on Earth, but Manifestation must be accepted, so that experience can bring the understandings. Form cannot be judged to be beneath Me. I am everything. When Spirits have shut Me out of their consciousness by their own limits, I have let them learn as long as possible and have interceded only when I have had to restore balance. Because I have not seemed to intercede lately, in ways that have been clearly apparent to those denying Me, these denials have seemed to prove their own judgments that I am not interested, don't exist, haven't any real powers, am beyond man or don't relate to man.

Judgments believed by the mind, and held in place by unmoving emotions, have drastically limited the channels open to Me to reach people in ways they can recognize as God. Refusal to recognize and accept Me has created a strong illusion of separation between Myself and most people on Earth. Many deny this separation, but the illusion is real enough for the ones experiencing it. Holding limits on Me does not allow you to see Me for what I am. This is not unlike worshipping a graven image.

Form is a manifestation of essence and must be aligned with essence in order to really manifest that essence. Confusion about

122

Form in the beginning caused many to deny their true Form in favor of another Form. In doing this, many had to deny some of their essence in order to take on another Form. Expression in Form has been imbalanced because of the imbalances between Spirit and Will. You can restore your true Form by aligning your Spirit and Will. True Form needs to return and will return. By taking the steps you can take to align with Me, you can make this process easier for yourself.

At one time, on Earth, I gave everyone who could accept it, human form, temporarily, to see if this would help them to work out confusion about Form. I have watched this closely, and I have clearly seen that even though I have restored the balance in Form numerous times, these Spirits have also continued to deny essence that is really theirs, and their Form is still trying to express this essence. Even though these Spirits have claimed that their problems were because they were different from others, giving them human form has not solved their problems. Many on Earth are not comfortable in human form, and yet, they asked Me for it and told Me that their true Form was not the Form they wanted to have. I have given these Spirits the maximum amount of time possible to give for experiencing a Form other than their true Form. The reality is that Spirits must now accept their true Form and realize that this is the Form in which they can best evolve.

Locking oneself into rigid Form, flowing through Form changes without realizing why, claiming that Form is all there is and claiming that Form is something to be transcended, are manifestations of some of the ways in which Form has been misunderstood, used and, thus, denied. Judgments about Form, and the accompanying emotional charge, are needing release along with the rest of your release so that Form can become more freely responsive, and your physical body will have the freedom to reflect your increasing self-acceptance.

I want to point out that some Spirits did not want their form to reflect their essence. These Spirits denied that their form did reflect their essence because they did not want to be seen for what they were. This denial of Form confused many others about form and essence, and they began to deny their true forms also. Some denied true form in an attempt to disguise themselves, some to aggrandize themselves and some in an attempt to diminish themselves. There are many emotions here.

One effect of these denials was to pressure Form toward becoming much more similar, and much less differentiated, than it is meant to be. This has been another attempt to limit Me by limiting My expression in Form. Many of the Spirits doing this claimed that I was trying to force essence into forms it did not want, or that I was punishing by forcing unwanted forms on Spirits who did not deserve it. While these points of view were certainly believed by many, all of Creation has free Will, whether the Spirits understand what this really means or have to learn it. Form has had a rigidity on Earth for quite some time, and this needs to heal now.

RIGHT USE OF WILL AS A HEALING POWER FOR YOURSELF AND EARTH

If you feel that you are holding too much to risk clearing yourself by starting with what has been given in this book, I suggest that you trust your own feelings here. Remember, though, that even small releases can help you, and if it is really too much for you, you can appeal to Me to bring you another way to heal yourself.

The pattern of increasing personal denial along with the denial of the Earth, itself, has been crossing the midpoint, which is why I must now intervene. Once denial has crossed the midpoint, once you have denied more than half of yourself, you have lost so much understanding and personal power that you must reclaim what you have lost, step by step, so that you are not misled by confusions the denials present. When you have denied more than half of yourself, your magnetic center is weaker than the denial, and denial has more power over your life than the rest of you has. This is the reality faced on Earth today. More than half of the Spirits on Earth have denied more than half of themselves.

Problems with keeping the full self together have been being handled by bringing forward only some of what needs be cleared at any one time. In terms of reincarnation, this has meant that people have been incarnating with only a part of themselves. See that increasing the holding patterns in the part that you have with you now can imperil your ability to clear. Aging and illness indicate that Body is in need of nourishment from My Loving Light. Death means that there is no other option, and for some people, this is going to be the case. It may be that Body cannot hold any more, or it may be that Earth is no longer that person's right place. For some, death means that not enough of the self came forward with them in this life, and they need to use this means to go and seek the rest of themselves in order to heal.

When you have stated intent to heal, whether you are able to recognize the form it comes in, or not, you can regard everything that comes your way as an opportunity to heal something. When you have cleared enough of what you have present with you, aligning with your full self is going to be necessary. This includes parts of you that you are not aware of yet. Some of you can draw these parts to you, some will need to go and join these parts and others will need to move in both of these ways.

Surrendering to your own Will and its progression is important, but this does not mean that the Will is supposed to control you. It means that the Will has been left so far behind that it needs focus to be able to catch up and come into present time. By no longer denying anything in yourself, your Spirit and your Will can find balance in your Heart. When the Will is freely able to respond to everything the Spirit has to suggest, it may, at times, appear that the Will does not want to accept some things from the Spirit. If the Spirit gives the Will as much time and understanding as the Will needs, and it still cannot align with the Spirit on some things, the Spirit needs to look at itself more fully. Do not make a judgment that something cannot happen if the Will cannot do it yet. It may not be the right time, or it may not be the right experience for you. When both Spirit and Will have unconditional acceptance of each other, each can fulfill its role. Heart then receives this balanced flow of energy and Body can freely manifest. This is the path of free Will and of unconditional love.

Denying and overriding and even deceiving, coercing and forcing the Will were instrumental in creating the original imbalances. When the Will, then, could not accept the experience it was having, the Spirit did not accept this pain from the Will. When Spirits didn't know what to do with the pain in their Will, many Spirits told their Wills they had to let go of these things without their Spirit having to receive it. The Will was not able to do this, and, then, felt it had to hold this until the Spirit would accept it. Most of this pain has been held from the very beginning.

When the Will's response was not accepted, the holding patterns that were established then, shutdown most of the Will. The overpowering of the Will has prevented it from having enough trust in Spirit to surrender easily to it. Because the Will felt that it could not come straight ahead and be accepted, it began to be manipulative, indirect or sideways in its approach to Spirit.

The Will needs the Spirit to give this held pain loving acceptance so that They can both gain trust.

Surrender means that you have unconditional acceptance. This is never achieved in any real way by overpowering something until it has to surrender. Neither Will nor Spirit is to be overpowered, and nothing is to be denied. Because anger often felt it couldn't be bothered with all this; it just wanted to do what it wanted to do, anger movement is going to be necessary. Where there are many old and deep denials, there may be resistance to the idea that manifesting this healing means you are going to have to go down first in order to bring these denials up and into present time.

Many have judged the physical self to be base and dense and have found themselves to be trapped in this. These Spirits began to break off from what they didn't love and leave their physical Body behind when they longed for other planes of existence and found that they could no longer speed up their physical Body and take it along.

Instead of denying how you feel about what the experience on Earth has been, realize that this denial is a way in which power has been being given to the very ones denying free Will on Earth. The fact that dissidents have been arrested, or worse, and that effective actions to curtail the overriding of free Will on Earth have, so far, met with so much denial is not reason to believe it will always be this way. If denial ends in the ones wishing to protect themselves and the Earth from being overridden, outer reality can shift.

The way to protect yourself and the Earth does not require that you do anything you don't want to do. Moving with your own internal process is going to be enough, if you really do it. This does not mean that your ability to act outwardly is going to be paralyzed. You are seeking to find balance, and imbalanced moves may be difficult to rectify. You can express the feelings you have about what is happening on Earth with yourself, to Me and with those you trust. Do not underestimate the power of this expression by judging or holding the judgment that expressing emotions does no good. By processing as much as you can before making any outer shifts in your life, ways can open to you, or become clear, in ways that were not apparent before.

Your internal alignment determines the power you have to get what you want. If, for example, from a place of partial alignment with yourself, you feel a need to ask Me to heal the Earth, I will respond to that request anyway because it is for the highest good of Earth. I do like to hear from you that you want this also, but I also want you to realize that this healing must happen in the way that will really bring the full healing that Earth needs.

If you ask Me to heal you and the Earth right now, it may appear that I am not answering your request if there is a time lag, or if you do not understand the form that this healing must take. This healing is a process of alignment. If you have denial in parts of yourself, you are not fully in touch with what could be holding back immediate response and instantaneous healing. Your healing must happen in the right way and at the right time. I must help you, and the Earth, to heal in the way that is appropriate. Even though healing is happening, you still need to process all of your responses to what is happening to you and around you. To be able to ask Me for something from a place of alignment, you need to know what all of you wants.

Original misunderstandings thought that pushing away everything that did not agree with what the conscious part wanted was the way to achieve alignment. As a result, most people have only part of themselves consciously present with them. Because these denials are parts of the self, they seek to return. When some parts of the self are not being given acceptance, they continue to seek access to the conscious awareness by drawing repeat patterns that reflect their presence. Because denial draws its own reflection, denials can draw experiences that are not what the conscious part thought it was creating. Your denials may be extensive, and buried enough, that they undermine the very things your conscious part wants to draw. In these places there is judgment instead of My Loving Light. Many of these denials are held in what has been called the subconscious, and to heal, you need to know what they are doing.

The way to heal yourself and the Earth is to end denial in yourself so that you have an alignment about what healing is for you and for the Earth. If part of you asks Me to heal you and the Earth, for example, and you hold in denial a part of you that is furious that things are they way they are, and that I haven't done this already, this denied part is not receptive to My help because it doesn't believe I am giving it. I cannot heal a part of you if it means lifting you away from other parts of you that are holding your denials. I cannot rescue you by lifting you away from a part of yourself, because you must take responsibility for your entire self. When you have denial present, healing often comes in the form of the experiences you need to help you recognize your denials. You must do your part as much as you can. If it is really too much for you, you may be lifted out temporarily, but you will still need to take responsibility later for what you haven't healed. This is why I am encouraging you to heal as much as you can now. If you feel this is a burdensome bother, let this anger surface and express until you are able to move to a place of deeper understanding with it.

Since healing must happen, everyone is getting what they need. When you have had disagreements with parts of yourself and, instead of finding alignment, they were denied participation with the rest of you, it can appear that they do not want the same things that you want. Then, one part cannot be answered without another part feeling denied. This is why so many people do not think they are getting what they want, but they are getting what they need, no matter how it looks. Since denials seek to gain acceptance and alignment by bringing themselves to your awareness, the more people have sought to keep denials away, the stronger the reflection has been getting. The fact of the matter is that when you have alignment, initially with your intent to heal and, then, with your full self, what you want and what you need are the same thing.

To heal the Earth, you need to heal yourself first. In ending your denials, you can tell Me everything you like and don't like about the reality in which you live and also how you want your reality to be. This can clarify your alignment with your right place, and is also important because it gives your healing parts a renewed vision to encourage them and an opportunity to express doubts and fears about whether this healing is possible or not.

Denial of Me has been involved here, too. So many people have believed that I am the God they think I am, rather than the God I am, that they have often limited My help to the ways in which they could imagine My help. Very often, help from Me is right there, and people haven't recognized it. Very often, I am right there, and people haven't recognized Me. You have the power to limit My Presence in your own life, but you do not have the power to limit Me. Along with aligning your own Spirit and Will, you need to align with Me. To do this, you need to release all judgments of what I am and what I am not. All the emotions that have been empowering these judgments also need to surface so they can shift. When you can really feel that I am a loving God, you will also be able to feel what is loving and what is not.

Right Use of Will offers an opportunity to accomplish more and also give oneself the opportunity to learn to come and go at Will from the physical plane again without having to use the birth/death approach. This can allow the Spirit to leave Earth with its entire self rather than with only the less dense levels of vibration and relieve people of much of the grief of separation when a loved one passes away. This alignment is necessary because the physical part of everyone is just as much a part of the Spirit as any other part. Body is the Divine Manifestation of Spirit, Will and Heart, and so, is the Fourth Aspect of My Light.

When you have aligned in this way, you will be able to ask Me to help you and the Earth, and know that I am. You will be able to ask Me for deeper understandings and to help you understand the needs of everything on Earth. You will be able to ask Me to restore the Earth to its full beauty, purity and ease of living. You will be able to hear Me and see Me at work there. You will be able to recognize it when I speak through people around you and when I do not. When you have alignment, you have agreement about what you want. This agreement allows it to happen because nothing in your energy field is in contradiction with your desire, and your desire is attracting it to you. When desire is aligned with Spirit, there is no problem in having your Heart's desire.

Spirit needs to inspire and guide, the Will needs to respond and their balanced interaction needs to select. However, the free and full response of the Will has been mostly missing, and I have seen that denial is why the Will has not been responding. Clearing this denial is going to allow true feelings to emerge, and true feelings can then tell Me how you would like your reality to be. I do not want to deny anything, and I won't, but you have the power to deny yourself. I am offering you this information as an opportunity to end your denial so that you can recognize, accept and feel gratitude for what you are being given. This recognition needs to be in all parts of you, not just the part that wants to tell Me that you already know this.

Healing the Earth is something that comes along with healing yourself more than you may be able to recognize in advance of the experience. If you are willing to take the path that leads to your own healing, you need only begin where you are, and let it unfold. You can tell Me anything you have in your consciousness and everything you want to have. While this is happening, you can feel Me drawing near as you open to receive My Loving Light.

STEPS TO HEALING
AND COMPLETE RECOVERY

Recognizing your own denials is the first step. Acknowledge every thought and feeling you would otherwise push away or ignore. I want to point out that 'positive thinking' is based on denial when it focuses on only parts of the self. Those parts get better and stronger, and the other parts get more denied. This is why so many have felt they need to discipline and otherwise pressure parts of the self. These denials are lost Will trying to press forward to gain expression and acceptance.

The next step is to release your judgments on these places in yourself and allow them to express themselves. Encourage them to tell you what they need and want.

The next step is reclaiming and integrating these denied parts of yourself. In so doing, you must not feel that this is just a mental exercise. You must accept everything that comes from any place in you and express it emotionally with yourself.

As your next step, seek to truly understand these denied parts. Feel into them to determine if this feels like it could be a part of you or not. Don't be too quick to disown things you don't like about yourself. Remember that denied parts will present as the judgments put against them. This may not be the essence of it once you take the judgments off of it and begin to accept it.

If your expression does feel like it could be a part of you, but is very sickened by its state of denial, you need to nurse it back to health in any way that you can. Talk to it. Encourage it to tell you its point of view. Accept its answers. Explain to it why you felt you had to deny it. Apologize to it. Ask its forgiveness. Most denials have been based in judgments of unlovingness according to your beliefs of what was loving and what was unloving at the time the judgments were made. When something that is being denied is judged to be unloving, it will appear that way by reflecting those judgments.

Negotiate a new relationship between these parts of yourself and the rest of you. Work on integrating these parts with the rest of you. Release any other judgments that come up, Allow these parts of yourself to be participants in your daily life. Accept their contributions to what you feel like doing.

If there continues to be no way you can come to peace with something here, you can ask My Light to put it in its right place. Then, let it go, and I will do this for you. If you feel a little ceremony is in order, do that, or ask Me for help in any way that feels right to you.

Another step you can take is to practice putting your consciousness into your body. You can breathe into your body and practice keeping your consciousness with your breath. Stay present with any places of blockage you find. Help it to surface, express and move whatever it has been holding. Body work can also help you find blockages you were not aware of. Reclaiming, integrating and healing lost Will involves going inside to where it is and bringing it up in vibration so that down can become up. To really heal, your entire body needs to become filled with the light of loving consciousness.

This is a process that is going to be ongoing for quite some time if you really get into it and seek to find all of your denials. If you feel you cannot spot all of your own denials, another step you can take is to let outer reality show them to you. If something is triggering to you it is likely you have lost Will involvement of some kind. This is something that has been a source of much confusion on Earth for a long time, but feeling it is going to straighten this out over time.

By looking at everything that is happening in the world you can see your own denials in outer reality. Let all of your feelings about it come up. Express them only with yourself at first and find out what they really are. When you feel ready, you can begin to start taking any action that you feel will improve your own situation. Notice everything you feel in relationship to taking action. Express those emotions. Do not push yourself to take action before you feel ready. If emotions come up at the idea of taking action, express those.

You can start with something simple that you feel you can do. For example, if someone is talking to you for longer than you want to listen, try telling this person you need to end the conversation. Say this right when you feel you want to end it, and don't give an untrue excuse for ending it. Say it gently before you feel angry about it.

Although this has not been considered polite in many circles, I want to point out that manners have so often been based in denial that many people have lost track of how they really feel and dare not act accordingly. The acceptance of true feelings will not need the guidance of 'manners' because attunement will be increasing. You will find this out by trying it.

If those around you do not accept this from you, another step you can take is to find in yourself what in you doesn't yet accept this and process that. Then, if there is still no acceptance for this, you may need to move on and find others who are not interested in denying each other in favor of externalized procedures. This is a form and essence misalignment.

The fear I see in people around this issue is that it is selfish and inconsiderate of others. To take it a step further, the fear is that societal structure will collapse and revert to chaos and anarchy if others do what they want to do. This is self-denial. I want to tell you that this is not going to happen. The issue here is a need for fear movement. If you are not doing what you want to do, it is not right for you to be doing it.

If you turn the tables on something that confuses you, you can more easily see it for what it is. For example, do you want someone to be talking or listening to you for longer they want to be? You can see how this feels to you and decide if you want to be doing this or not. If it would not feel good to you to be the receiver of what you are doing, then, don't do it.

The only place you can start is where you really are. Since so much personal power has been denied and subsequently lost, starting with simple things and going on from there is going to be an ongoing process of reclaiming your personal power. Power has become such a nasty word on Earth right now, but who has most of it? Isn't it the ones imparting to you that you should not have any? They have your denied power to work with.

Spirits are not meant to overpower one another. At present, personal power is seriously imbalanced on Earth, yet you can only be overpowered by others if you have given up some of your own power that they can, then, use against you. The imbalance of power through guilt and intimidation of various kinds took place step by step, and you will need to restore the balance step by step. What are your judgments against power?

The Spirits that have an interest in overpowering others can only increase their power by getting others to abdicate their power. It is a powerful illusion; increasing power by diminishing others. This has been happening for such a long time on Earth that many do not believe they have power over their own lives any more. In general, birth to death is regulated. Think of everything you believe you have to do just to be able to go on living on Earth.

This is not the way it is meant to be. Everything on Earth is meant to be free, abundant and hospitable. No one is meant to do what he/she doesn't want to do to have food and shelter. Misunderstandings about denial changed this.

Overpowering does not need to happen between parents and children, either. Children need an opportunity to develop their own responses to situations, and learn to choose accordingly. Guidance is one thing. Telling children what to think and feel is another. Right Use of Will is for all ages.

If parents are not meaning to interfere with the Free Will of their children, but do not really understand it, let Me say this: It does not mean letting the children run over you. Do not deny yourselves in favor of the children and do not deny the children in favor of yourselves. This is a balance that acknowledges that the parents learn from the children as well as the children learning from their parents.

If the children's behavior doesn't make sense to you as the parent and they are not harming anyone, support them and let them learn. Protect them while they are learning. This is Right Use of Will because you are not requiring them to see everything your way, but are letting them learn from their own experiences.

The reason I say this is because any understandings at all will increase the light and make further understandings possible. Only total refusal to accept anything at all will keep you in darkness. Trying to keep others where you are is not Right Use of Will. If children are seeing things that you are not yet seeing, rest assured that they need to see them and be allowed to experience what they need to experience to learn what they need to learn. Support them in this and encourage them to communicate with you about it.

Male or female, do not shame them for having fear. Fear can be such a helpful caution. Protecting children from danger is necessary, and intuition may say there is danger ahead, but protecting them from the possible danger you see them as encountering is imposing your perceptions onto them.

For example, when a child climbs, rather than run over there screaming "Get down before you fall," be there and support the child in his/her efforts. Notice it if you have converted your fear to anger in this situation.

This recognition of children's growing abilities will support their confidence and self-acceptance. As children grow they will become more and more able to recognize their own potentials and their potential dangers. Then, the job of protecting them can become easier and easier and involve less limitations for all of you. If your own fear is too great to allow this kind of approach, you can work with your own fears and try not to give them to your child.

By the time the children are ready to leave home they won't have to feel that they must leave to get free of constrictions and restrictions nor become reactionary to limitations and controls on their behavior.

If the situation has not been as described here, it can still begin. Starting where you are is the only point for beginning. Seeing that the child and the parents are together to learn from each other and not just the child from the parents will accelerate the growth. Chances are that feelings will need some time to reach the understandings needed. Allow time to show you what you need to see.

The process of ending your denial and expanding into your full consciousness and personal power is not simple, but neither is it too difficult for you to do. Compared to how long it's been going in the opposite direction, this can happen relatively quickly if you really dedicate yourself to it. The first thing you will notice as you release your emotional blockages is a greater ease with yourself. Then, you will begin feeling things you didn't know you felt. Your seeing and hearing will expand, and you will begin to get information from seeing, hearing and feeling that you were not aware of before. The appearance of your body will begin to change. This will all be gradual at first, but will increase as you can handle it. If you want to, you can ask Me to help you with all of this. Your Spirit can speak directly to you when you can accept it.

If you seriously work on this process, and it does not seem to work for you, you need to find denials you have not recognized yet. You may need to move slower or it may not be right time for you. Process whatever you can and whatever you are triggered into and healing will come one way or another. Healing yourself has to succeed if you have strong intent.

Healing is what I want for Earth now, not doomsday as some people say. If you do not recognize the process of healing, you may think it is doomsday. I feel the Wills on Earth calling for the release of pain, and I am now responding.

In processing this you need to trust your feelings extensively. In doing this do not judge your feelings any more than they have been judged already. Try it out and see if it feels better than what you were doing before. Healing in the entire sense of the word is going to heal everything in you, and healing in entirety is going to have a transformative effect on your reality.

INTIMIDATING FORM

Form has intimidated many on Earth because it has not been understood. If you look around, there seems to be a whole world full of intimidating form that appears to have power over you to tell you how you have to live, what you have to do and even how you are to think and feel. I could make a long list here, but I will only list areas that have overridden nearly everyone's free Will and had the power to force compliance.

Laws, rules and regulations are not necessary in a society of free Will, and they are not valid in a society that is in support of freeing the Will unless they have the purpose of protecting people from being overridden by others, no matter who they may be. Many laws that appeared to start out this way have become imprisoning because of the ways in which they have been applied. Laws should really be guidelines to preserve the balance points in society. Enforcing laws is another intimidating form. Society will exist without any law enforcement if it is a valid society. Compulsory education has become another intimidating form to some, as well as having to have formal education to be considered "qualified" and, then, also to have to pay the cost of it or have your innate knowing shut out. Family pressure can be another intimidating form and, for many, is the first place to begin understanding the presence of intimidating form in your life.

Another intimidating form is the idea of land ownership and national borders. Yet another intimidating form is the belief that you have to buy something or pay rent all of your life to have any place to live on Earth. Added to that is the idea that you must have a job to pay for it and also pay taxes forever. Another intimidating form that needs mention is the frequently repeated admonition that nobody owes you anything, but, meanwhile, you are always owing.

Industry is another intimidating form. The idea that large companies are needed to manufacture the things needed in everyday life is an intimidating form that has, itself, been manufactured. Relative to this, I am wondering how many pieces of plastic people are going to exchange for money without realizing that they're not getting anything real for their money or their labors. Instead of leaving a legacy of beautiful and lasting creativity that can be handed down, the current legacy is one of deterioration and residual pollutants.

The establishment of a military in every nation is another intimidating form that has convinced many people of its necessity and power. Industry and the military present as though they expect people to continue living on Earth and, yet, they have both treated the Earth as something they plan to discard in the near future. I will not allow this, however. Instead, they are going to be removed and put in their right place.

Form is a reflection of the consciousness it holds. Acid rain and other chemical pollutants, as well as radioactivity, have been reflecting denied death wishes held by many people on Earth toward themselves and toward Creation. The way Earth has been handled has made these intimidating forms appear to be both very overwhelming and unchangeable. One intimidating form has been compounded by another and another and leveraged by other intimidating forms, and has created a massive façade of intimidating form. These intimidating forms are a temporary reality, and yet, they have become so prominent and so layered in with so much conditioning, that many people have not been able to recognize them as a false reality that is based in denial. It is denial that has enabled and empowered and, also, made necessary, all of these intimidating forms.

Intimidating form promotes the appearance of a rigidity that is not individually responsive, but imposes a set form on all people. Even though protests have brought many attempts to make rules that are supposed to apply to different sets of people, it still remains an externalized agenda, set in place by people who are not present in the moment. It has been externalized to an outer authority that has awarded itself power over you and what happens in your life. It is not a person feeling another person and deciding how they can help. It is ritualized and divested of subjectivity, which is a form of Will denial.

There are many judgments against the self here. One prominent example is: I cannot trust myself to manage my life. Release of this judgment does not mean that you must know everything yourself. Being told what to do by an outer voice of "authority" is different than seeking helpful advice and arriving at decisions about how to proceed.

Religions are another intimidating form that has given rules and told people to abdicate their Will in favor of My Will.

Religions have then promoted their own point of view and called it My Will. It is not possible to find Me there, because guilt is most of the presence; guilt that has been passed off as love. Religions have given form to something I said or did in the past as though this is what is also right for any similar situation that has occurred since then. Sometimes this is applicable, and sometimes it is not. The giving of these teachings as though they are universal laws to remain unchanged forever has not been opening receptivity to the change and evolution of the living God that I am. For example, interpretations of the scripture that man shall not spill his seed upon the ground, has led to further fragmentation, a loss of freedoms, an increase in regulations and a loss of the Earth's right to renewing, nurturing and uplifting, wild and free places.

Quality of life is what makes life worth living. When parents have children they do not fully want, it has been draining to the parents, and the Will denial involved has resulted in the fragmentation that is now most people. Lack of free movement in the Will has been giving rise to all of these forms that have become so intimidating, but saying this does not mean that I am promoting change for the sake of change, or the denial patterns of promoting change for increased sales or as a distraction from boredom.

I hear the complaint on Earth: If I recover myself, I still have to live on Earth and the more sensitive I get, the harder it is to handle what is happening. I want to reassure you here. Everything that has been attempted on Earth, so far, has had denial present in it. In recovering lost sensitivities, protect them in any way you feel you need to, but also give them emotional expression so that you do not repeat your original patterns of denial. By moving with whatever you can, you can end your own denials. Ending your own denials is going to affect everything around you, but because of the way these denials were put in place, things can look and feel worse before they get better.

I do not want to tell you any more, now, about how it is going to be later, because fixing on images according to the level of understanding you have now can prevent you from attaining the movement necessary. What you need to know, now, is that guilt, unlovingness and denial has had more presence than My Loving Light on Earth. Much denial of the Will has been based in the belief that acting from guilt and self-denial was being loving toward others. This has meant that the Will has not been allowed to move in many of the ways the Will wants and needs to move.

A judgment here has been that the Will is not loving, when, in actuality, it is guilt that is not loving. Love does not seek self-denial.

Intimidating form on Earth is a reflection of denial and guilt. Whether you understand My Light on this, yet, or not, if you allow movement in your Will, you can gain the understandings as you go along, however, the presence of denial and guilt on Earth has not wanted to allow this movement because it has been holding the judgments against it. To get the changes you need in the intimidating form around you that has said you cannot do and say as you want, you need to heal this lost Will in yourself first.

This caution is necessary for you, at least until you know more about what you are doing. Form intimidates only those over whom it has power. Movement within yourself will show you how you have been empowering these intimidating forms with your own self-denial. So, take My caution seriously here. Advancing outwardly is not going to be successful for you unless you have done the inner movement first. If you meet what feels like impenetrable resistance, retreat and process whatever has been triggered. Later, you can try again.

What is happening on Earth now can help you to recognize your own denials. You can do this most easily by giving in to your emotions first and analyzing it later. Be assured that nothing is going to happen to you unless it is necessary to help you clear your own denials. Healing is what I have in mind for Earth right now, although, if you cannot recognize the process of healing, you may think it is doomsday.

I feel the Wills on Earth calling for release of their pain, and I am responding. If you have the intent and manifest your intent by really doing this process, healing yourself has to succeed, no matter what form it takes. In doing this, you need to trust your feelings extensively. Accept whatever your feelings have to offer, and trust that your Will has a progression of unfoldment. Instead of trying to manage, direct, pressure or force; allow it. Try not to judge your feelings any more than you already have. Release all the judgments you have been holding on yourself that you can. Healing in the entire sense is going to heal everything in you, and healing yourself entirely is going to have a transformative effect on your reality.

In saying this, I do not mean that there is hope at the end of a long struggle. I mean that this can happen now. You do not have to heal everything in sight immediately. You only need to find your own denials, accept them and have intent to heal them as soon as you can. If you have been convinced that magic is deception or is evil and not a part of Me, just try what I have presented here and see what happens on Earth.

I will not say much more now, except that I have completed the teaching for this book, and I know you can do it. I have chosen not to go into depth in any one area because I see how many people already have parts of this information, and also, how many people are not, yet, ready for more. Putting the parts together is My purpose here. In doing that, I have needed to point out what has been holding the parts separate from each other. In healing yourself, look carefully at everything that has held you apart from your full self and from others. This is where emotional blockages and old judgments are held, and this is where denial hides. These are holes in the energy field that have to heal and can be healed without scars if they are healed completely.

I have seen already that Earth has to heal now. I have already seen that Earth can heal now. I have already seen that many people on Earth need to heal now, and I have seen that many people can heal now. I hear the call from many who want to hear from Me directly, and I do speak to a number of people on Earth. People hear from Me what they are ready to accept. Many people who hear Me have not realized it is Me speaking to them. Others have wanted to hear from Me and have thought that they did when they did not. How to tell the difference between My Loving Light and other voices is the question here. You must know your own intent and your own Heart. The more you clear your own Will, the more it can be felt to be My guiding presence or not. You can help yourself by going slowly here and feeling into it.

I am everything, and I am in all places in one form or another. I love all of My Spirits, and I want to give them all what they want and need. If I am not feeling good to you in this form, then this is not the right form for you at this time. If you need to relate to Me differently, you will find the image you need. I hold no judgment or denial here. I will just put you in the place where you can receive Me in the way that you want to receive Me. I have only healing in mind here, and I want you to know that it is entirely possible to heal Earth in the coming years. I will do it, and you can help Me by healing as much of yourself as you can. I will help anyone who needs My help in any way in which they can receive Me if I am asked to be present.

The more you open to yourself and the more of yourself you receive into your own love, the more you can open to Me and increase your own light on Earth. Earth has My Unlimited Love, and the more you open to Me, the more My Light will increase within you and on Earth. I end now with one of My favorite endings.

Amen

RIGHT USE OF WILL
Healing and Evolving the Emotional Body
is the first in a series of books
channelled by Ceanne DeRohan

The other books are:
ORIGINAL CAUSE I
The Unseen Role of Denial
ORIGINAL CAUSE II
The Reflection Lost Will Has to Give
EARTH SPELL
The Loss of Consciousness on Earth
HEART SONG
Vibrating Heartlessness to Let Heart In
LAND OF PAN
The Loss of Power and Magic on Earth
IMPRINTING
The Healing of the Chakras
INDIGO
The Search for
True Understanding and Balance

These books need to be read in order. Getting ready for the sequels involves moving along with the material in Right Use of Will enough to know if this information is right for you.

These books let you know your Original Cause by helping you access belief systems lost in the subconscious long ago, yet influencing our lives every day.

We appreciate it that you have bought this book. If you are interested in other books and cannot get them through your local store, you can get ordering information by using the ISBN for Right Use of Will in Books in Print or on the web at www. rightuseof will.com. Thank you.

FOUR WINDS PUBLICATIONS

ISBN 978-1-929113-00-2

Made in the USA
Coppell, TX
22 October 2023

23208654R00089